The Curious

Research by family doctors in Canada

in the early years

* * * * * * * *

Dr. Bill Falk

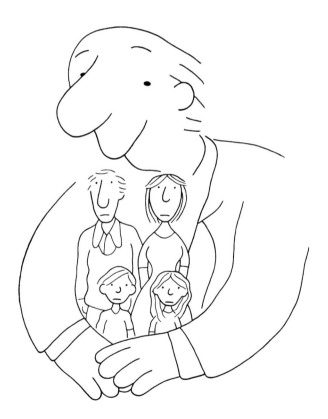

If you have any comment or additions, contact the author at:

Address: 308 - 2278 James White Boulevard
               Sidney, B.C., Canada
               V8L 1Z4
Phone: (250) 655-0024
Fax: (250) 655-0018
E-mail: wafme@home.com

National Library of Canada Cataloguing in Publication Data

Falk, William Andre, 1924-
  The curious family doctor

Includes index.
  ISBN 1-55212-777-X

  1. Family medicine--Research--History. I. Title.
R850.F35 2001   610'.7   C2001-911241-6

TRAFFORD

This book was published *on-demand* in cooperation with Trafford Publishing.
On-demand publishing is a unique process and service of making a book available for retail sale to the public taking advantage of on-demand manufacturing and Internet marketing.
On-demand publishing includes promotions, retail sales, manufacturing, order fulfilment, accounting and collecting royalties on behalf of the author.

Suite 6E, 2333 Government St., Victoria, B.C. V8T 4P4, CANADA
Phone   250-383-6864   Toll-free   1-888-232-4444 (Canada & US)
Fax   250-383-6804   E-mail   sales@trafford.com
Web site   www.trafford.com TRAFFORD PUBLISHING IS A DIVISION OF TRAFFORD HOLDINGS LTD.
Trafford Catalogue #01-0177 www.trafford.com/robots/01-0177.html

  10   9   8   7   6   5   4   3

Acknowledgements

Writing about personal experiences and attitudes imposes a responsibility on the author to aim for accuracy and reasonable completeness. My motivation has been helped by the late Dr. John Garson, who read the earliest version and made helpful comments and suggestions for inclusion. Dr. Bob Westbury has always been encouraging and felt that this effort was worth continuing after a look at a draft copy.

With a focus on family medicine, it was natural for my own family to be involved. Our daughter, Andrea, a whiz on the Macintosh computer, helped me through many times when the computer would not recognize my orders. Her spouse, Gilbert, expanded our hardware capacity into the mega range, and helped it to recover from its ailments. Elder son Bruce, a computer programmer (not a Macintosh fan) also helped to sort out problems. Younger son Graham, a born artist, drew some impressions of the medical scene, at the age of fourteen. Molly, my wife of many years, was immensely helpful with proof-reading, suggestions re content and wording, taking and placing pictures and especially with continuing motivational encouragement – "are you going to finish your book today?" - she really should be named as co-author.

Without the interest and help of these supporters, and the expert help at Trafford Publishing, it would have taken even longer to get to the stage where the line must be drawn, even while knowing that much more detail should have been included.

To

Dr. Jim Collyer

1933 – 1989

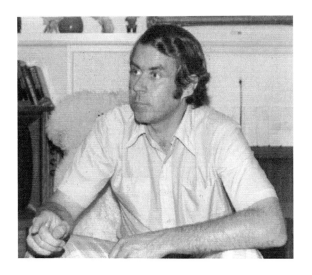

who inspired so many family doctors by his example as a
researcher, a teacher and a person

The Curious Family Doctor

Table of contents

Foreword

In the eighties and nineties, there was a progressive increase in research in family medicine, to the point where it is difficult to keep track of it. This increase has been based on a foundation laid by many general practitioners who saw the need and tried to meet it, or who simply tried to satisfy their own curiosity. This book is written to bring together scattered records of studies done by the pioneers, mainly limited to the third quarter of the twentieth century. It does not claim to be complete, but at least provides a record of much of the early work, and as such is archival.

One of the first principles learned in the development of a research program is to define your terms. It is vital to define the concept of general practice or family medicine, so that we all know what we are talking about. The general practitioner (or G.P.) has long been known as the family doctor, and still is in countries which have retained the term. The family physician label was adopted in 1967 by the College of Family Physicians of Canada, and shortly afterwards by the American Academy of Family Physicians, in response to a perceived need to define an area of expertise as departments of family medicine were starting up in the medical schools. For the purpose of this book, as in practice, the terms 'general practitioner', 'family physician' or 'family doctor' are interchangeable.

What is general practice?

General practice covers the full gamut of medical care, and in some isolated areas a bit of dental and veterinary care. The G.P. is ideally the first point of contact with the medical system, dealing with undifferentiated illness often in the early stages. The G.P. can deal with problems in any diagnostic category, at any stage, and in any age group. Various studies have shown that from 80 to 90 percent of problems can be managed completely, and the rest will require consultation or action by specialists. The percentage requiring consultation varies according to personal abilities, geographic location, supply of specialists, hospital regulations and pressure from patients.

The natural history of disease can be followed from the earliest sign of illness to the final result, especially in established practices which can cover many decades. There is usually some intervention in most diseases, so that the evaluation of the results of treatment becomes relevant.

Research Base

Medical schools had been staffed mostly by specialists, who provided most of the teaching of medical students and interns. Dr. Kerr White displayed a diagram to show the use of various medical resources by the population (White, K., 1961). Of 1,000 adults (aged 16 and over), about 750 reported one or more illnesses during a month. Of these, about 250 consulted a physician at least once during the month. Of these, about 9 required hospital care. About 5 were referred to another physician, of which one was referred to a university medical centre. Therefore much of the teaching of medical students involved $1/1,000^{th}$ of the population, most of whom did not have problems dealt with frequently by family doctors.

There have been major changes in the medical and political fields since Dr. White's study in 1957-1959 in North Carolina and Great Britain. Admission to hospital is less available, because of the closing of many hospitals and the increase in the use of outpatient surgery services. The role of general practitioners in the hospital has been reduced so that students have less contact with them except in the family medicine residency programs. The research base in hospitals is restricted to a different population than is seen in general practice.

In the late sixties and early seventies there was a great surge of interest and activity in family medicine research in Canada. This interest was largely the result of pioneering work done by individuals and committees who saw the potential value of such research before it became a major theme of the College of Family Physicians of Canada, or of most departments of family medicine in our teaching centres.

Hurdles

One of the biggest problems facing the private general practitioner who developed an interest in research was to fit it in with fulltime practice responsibilities. Smaller projects could be handled, because of the interest and the relatively small cost in time and money. Larger projects might require support from a granting agency, which would pay only out-of-pocket expenses but nothing for the time of the principal investigator. It seemed that there were few allowances for a researcher who was not at least partly supported by a salary. Later, when university departments began to develop research programs in family practice, for some faculty members the time for research was protected as part of the working time, or even a requirement.

An early account of GP research

In 1979, a valuable account of the early years of general practice research in Canada was given by David Woods, in his book about the first twenty-five years of the College of Family Physicians, "Strength in Study" (Woods, D., 1979). He cited a 1971 report in the Practitioner by Dr. Michael Livingston (Livingston, M., 1971), who found that only fifteen Canadian family doctors had contributed original observations to the literature during the previous two decades. In spite of Dr. Livingston's list being short, it shows that there was an active interest in research before there was a major effort by the College of General Practice of Canada or medical schools to encourage and support it. However, even this short list included more case reports and observations than organized research projects.

In writing this book, I feel qualified mainly as an admiring observer of many of the early participants in family practice research, as well as having some part in its development by doing studies in my own practice and working with various research committees. I have also been impressed by the valuable work done in other countries and will include some details which have a direct bearing on the progress of our work in Canada. Examples of their studies, and personal contact with many of their researchers, helped to increase the motivation of family doctors in Canada and the feeling that the efforts to do research were important.

Chapter 1

Inspiration and motivation

In 1964, Dr. Robin Pinsent from Birmingham, England, visited Montreal. It was for the combined meeting of the College of General Practice of Canada, in its Annual Scientific Assembly, and the first meeting of the international group which was to become WONCA (World Organization of National Colleges and Academies of General/Family Practice). Dr. Pinsent set up a display by the escalators in the Queen Elizabeth Hotel, where registrants passed on their way to and from the meeting rooms. They could see examples of recording systems in use in Britain and were exposed to his infectious enthusiasm for research. Dr. Pinsent continued to encourage the Canadian work by mail and by occasional contacts at Canadian and international meetings, even after his retirement to Devon.

When the College's National Research Committee started its series of workshops for training general practitioners in research methods, it was natural to turn to the known experts in Britain for help. At the first national research meeting, held at the University of Western Ontario (Western), January 17-18, 1969, keynote speakers were <u>Dr. Ian Watson and Dr. Ian McWhinney.</u>

Dr. Watson practised in the village of Peaslake, Surrey. He had been involved in research when young, seeing his father's work on malaria research in southeast Asia. Ian Watson ran the Epidemic Observation Unit (E.O.U.), described below. This very useful work was done at little expense in his surgery, attached to his home, with the aid of his practice secretary. The E.O.U. was the inspiration for the National Recording Service (NaReS) in Canada.

Dr. Ian McWhinney had worked in a group practice in Stratford-upon-Avon in England before joining the Faculty of Medicine at the University of Western Ontario in 1968. While in England, he published a book on *'The Early*

Signs of Illness', a practical guide for the young practitioner (McWhinney, I.L., 1964). At the Subdepartment of Family Medicine he promoted a research interest, and developed a research program which was considered to be the best in Canada, and which has remained in the top rank with a continuing major commitment. During the early seventies, he invited experienced researchers to enrich the program.

Dr. Donald Crombie, from the Birmingham Research Unit of the Royal College of General Practitioners, spent one year as a visiting professor. He was also supported for three months by The College, to allow him to accept invitations from provincial research committees to consult with them or to contribute to workshops. His first workshop was in January, 1973, at Harrison Hot Springs, B.C. Others were held at Halifax, Nova Scotia and Sackville, New Brunswick.

Similarly, Dr. Bent Guttorm Bentsen from Norway came for a year as visiting professor, and later returned to head the first family practice program in Norway, at Trondheim. Dr. Bentsen had done a major study of general practice in Norway, reported in his book *'Illness and General Practice'* (Bentsen, B.G., 1970).

Other visitors who were involved with the College's workshops are mentioned in Chapter Four.

The Nuffield Foundation

The work of the Royal College of General Practitioners (RCGP) was recognized by the Nuffield Foundation in Britain, which has provided many fellowships in a variety of fields, to enable individuals from commonwealth countries to travel to meet colleagues with similar interests. The series of Commonwealth Travelling Fellowships for general practitioners provided three fellowships per year over a twelve-year period. They allowed fellows to travel to other commonwealth countries and the U.S.A. to meet general practitioners and their organizations or medical facilities. Each year there were two fellows chosen in Britain and one in the commonwealth, rotating through Australia, New Zealand and Canada. Study topics were selected by applicants, who were nominated by their own colleges according to the relevance of their plans. The final choice was made by the RCGP from the short list submitted. Conditions for the fellowship were generous, providing for a six-month tour with travel costs paid and a daily allowance. It also provided funds to help support a locum to maintain the practice during the time away. Any extra costs were borne by the traveller, mainly the travel and accommodation needed for any extra persons or side trips.

At the 1964 meeting in Montreal, where Dr. Pinsent attracted potential research workers, I also happened to meet two Australians who made a difference. Dr. Ben Adsett, from Brisbane in Queensland, was the 1964 Nuffield Travelling Fellow, looking at the methods in the U.K., Canada and the U.S.A. for providing continuing education for general practitioners. On his return to Australia he represented the Australian College of General Practitioners (ACGP) in its education program. Dr. Clifford Jungfer, from Adelaide in South Australia, was a founding member of the ACGP and a continuing contributor to its progress.

Encouraged by Drs. Adsett and Jungfer, I thought that the fellowship could provide a great opportunity to learn more about general practice research.

The terms of the fellowship required that the candidate's spouse should go for at least three months. Molly had rather casually agreed to go, as I was filling out the form, although I had the feeling that she really did not expect to go. At that time neither of us could have predicted where our decision would take us. Not until the dream became a reality did we find that the only acceptable way to provide for our three children (Graham, aged 8, Andrea at 10 and Bruce at 12) was to take them along for the first three months. We became a 'close' family for those three months, especially when travelling around Britain in a Morris Minor, or camping in a sixteen-foot caravan at Gower Point near Swansea (courtesy of Dr. W.O. Williams) or all five in one room in a pensionat in Copenhagen. I have often thought

3

about what an imposition it was to arrive with three children, but we did enjoy some memorable times with our hosts, and still greatly appreciate their hospitality. Since then we have welcomed any chance to reciprocate when medical travellers have come through, especially if children are included.

Travels in Britain

When the Nuffield Fellowship was awarded to me in 1965, I followed the advice and help given by Dr. Robin Pinsent. Through him, I met many active family practice research workers and learned of many of the projects they had completed or which were in progress.

One of the best examples of original work was done by <u>Dr. William Pickles</u> in the isolated village of Aysgarth, in Yorkshire, England. He knew all the people in his area, as well as their cats and dogs. He recorded all cases of infectious disease in his community, simply by marking their occurrence on squared graph paper, using different colours for each of the diseases encountered. The time and expense involved were relatively little, in relation to the value of the results, which provided the material for his book 'Epidemiology in a Country Practice' (Pickles, W.N., 1949). He was able to follow the course of an epidemic, and sometimes trace it to its original source outside his area. In following his routine, he made original observations on the epidemiology of catarrhal jaundice (hepatitis) which were important enough to be published in the Lancet (Pickles, W.N., 1939). We had the good luck, through Dr. Bill Foster in Leeds (who later migrated to Victoria, B.C.), to visit Dr. Pickles in his village home. He was retired and in his eighties but still mentally alert. The copy of his unique book, which he autographed and gave to me, has sadly disappeared from my library.

Dr. Pickles had a great influence on the development of general practice in Britain, through his research and as the first president of the Royal College of General Practitioners in 1952. He is still honoured by the annual Pickles Memorial

Oration, given by a speaker chosen for achievement in general practice. A biography of Dr. Pickles was written by Dr. John Pemberton, giving details of his practice, his many honours and his lectures to general practitioners and epidemiologists in many countries (Pemberton, J., 1970).

According to Pemberton, Dr. Pickles had been inspired by the book by Dr. James McKenzie (McKenzie, J., 1916), who had practised in the town of Burnley in Lancashire, not far from Aysgarth. In his nearly thirty years of general practice, McKenzie had been interested in the heart and its rhythms to the point where he invented a pulse-recording system which has developed into our modern electrocardiograph.

James McKenzie said:
"As a result of my experience … I assert with confidence that medicine will make but halting progress, while whole fields essential to the progress of medicine will remain unexplored, until the general practitioner takes his place as an investigator."

Britain was the world leader in general practice research, where the pioneers have led the way. In 1952 the College of General Practitioners was formed and gave a great stimulus to the members interested in research. In 1965, the Records and Statistical Unit was well-established in Birmingham, with Dr. Robin (R.J.F.H.) Pinsent as Research Advisor. This unit was supported by the Nuffield Provincial Hospitals Trust, which seemed to appreciate the importance of general practice in the health care of the country.

The Research Committee of Council, chaired by Dr. Donald Crombie of Birmingham, provided direction but delegated authority to units and working parties for most of the projects supported by the RCGP (the 'Royal' label was added to the name in 1962). Many useful reports had been published as supplements to the journal of the RCGP. The committee's research register included more than 750 members interested in or participating in research. Dr. Crombie was an early contributor, with a one-year study of the use of time in general practice (Crombie, D.L., 1956).

Guided by advice and arrangements by Dr. Pinsent, I visited many of the research practices, units and individuals, too many to include in this book which is intended to show examples of what has been done.

Epidemic Observation Unit

This unique service was run by <u>Dr. G.I.Watson</u> in his surgery in Peaslake, Surrey. About fifty recorders sent him postcards weekly, listing patients they had seen during the previous week with the conditions currently under study. Dr. Watson and his secretary collated results promptly and circulated them to the College and the government. This system provided early warning of epidemics or conditions of interest before the routine public health announcements were available. Usually there were three or four topics. Examples were: severe adult chickenpox, survivors of childhood cancer, rubella, leukemia, febrile convulsions, early symptoms of cancer. When there were enough reports on a topic, or it was no longer timely, another would take its place on the cards.

Congenital Abnormalities Survey

Before the government collected data about defects noted at birth, the RCGP maintained a register of congenital abnormalities, recorded by <u>Dr. Basil Slater</u>. The findings were used in conjunction with the Outcome of Pregnancy Survey. They showed seasonal variation in some types of abnormality.

Cancer Study Group

<u>Dr. Ian McWhinney</u> (1964 Nuffield Travelling Fellow), in a series of one hundred patients, had noted discrepancies between presenting symptoms described as common in textbooks and those in his patients. He set up a larger prospective study to collect data on the earliest symptoms of suspected cancer, with follow-up to show which patients actually developed cancer. For five years new diagnoses of cancer were recorded, in a group practice with 6,681 patients at the start and 7,765 at the end, plus nearly 200 private patients.

There were 98 new diagnoses of cancer, including 43 patients over the age of 70. The practice had fewer patients over 50 than the general population. An unexpected finding was that cough was an uncommon symptom in cancer of the lung (McWhinney, I.R., 1962).

The Content of Practice
Surveys were underway in Wales by Dr. W.O. Williams (Williams, W.O., 1964) and in southwest England by Dr. H.J. Wright (Wright, H.J., 1968) to collect data from a large number of practices for one week in each three-month period of the year. There had already been a baseline study of morbidity over the year in 106 practices in 1955, which served as a comparison for future studies.

Tamar Valley Study
The town of Tavistock in Devon was served by an unusual water supply, with separate sources for each of three areas of the town. Dr. Robin Pinsent had a special interest, as his father had developed cancer while living there. It seemed obvious that the water supply must be suspected as a cause of cancer, because of distribution of cases in the town. Despite Dr. Pinsent's expert ability and motivation to prove cause and effect, no proof was found, but he did learn about the difficulty of environmental studies (Records and Statistics Unit, 1966). He had an ally in his interest in environmental studies – Dr. Harry Warren, Professor of Geology at the University of British Columbia. Dr. Warrren became a supporter of the research committee of the B.C. Chapter of The College in trying to develop a project to study the effects of trace elements.

Outcome of pregnancy
A prospective study by Dr. Donald Crombie involved a large number of patients from practices throughout Britain. Details were recorded from the earliest stages of pregnancy, including medications, illnesses and infections in other members of the family, also possible factors in the pre-conception period.

Farmer's lung

In 1957, <u>Dr. Howard Staines</u> of Callington, Cornwall, conducted a survey of farmer's lung in the United Kingdom, finding 444 cases, with a reponse rate of 36% of general practitioners. Wales and Southeast Anglia had the most cases (Staines, F.H., 1961).

Virology

<u>Dr. Edgar Hope-Simpson</u> of Cirencester, near the Cotswolds in England, was supported by the Medical Research Council to maintain a virus laboratory on his practice premises. With a long-term interest in epidemiology, he had shown by epidemiologic methods that herpes zoster and chickenpox were caused by the same virus, before there was laboratory proof (Hope-Simpson, R.E., 1954 and 1963).

Practice profile

<u>Dr. John Fry</u> in Beckenham, Kent, kept track of his patients on index cards. He described his simple but effective methods, which could be used in any practice (Fry, J., 1956). A regular contributor to journals and academic meetings, he published results from his practice in a series of papers following the development of his practice through the years (Fry, J., 1952, 1957, 1964) and then a book about the natural history of common diseases (Fry, J., 1966). He also was a member of the Council of the RCGP and was often invited overseas to speak to family doctors.

An early practice study

Near the heart of London, <u>Drs. John and Elizabeth Horder</u> recorded 2,000 consecutive cases to show the variety of diagnoses made in summer and in winter. In a separate group of 300 patients they recorded the amount and type of illness which was treated by the family doctor, the number of patients going directly to the hospital or a specialist, and the amount of illness not treated by any medical service. In a diagram showing the relative proportions, there were 190 first consultations with the family doctor, 17 with other agencies, and 514 managed by the patient or family (Horder,

J. & E., 1954). The practice was in a highly-populated area, where the daily round of house calls could be made on foot.

Long term study with follow-up

Another pioneer was <u>Dr. Keith Hodgkin</u> of Redcar, Yorkshire, who kept records on patients seen during medical school, hospital training, and practice. The long-term record helped him to write a unique book 'Towards Earlier Diagnosis' (Hodgkin, K., 1963, evolving to a fifth edition in 1985). He showed the probability of various diseases developing after initial symptoms, such as abdominal pain, followed to a final diagnosis. He also calculated the incidence and prevalence of all the common diseases, and of the uncommon but important ones. In Canada, he became the Professor of Family Medicine at Memorial University in St. Johns, Newfoundland. From there, he became a frequent contributor to family medicine scientific sessions across the country. His practical, simple and humourous talks were understood and appreciated by his audiences, who had too often been subjected to formal talks and inadequate audio-visual presentations.

Travels in Europe

Although the primary purpose of the Nuffield tour was to visit general practitioners in the Commonwealth, it seemed appropriate to make contacts in countries which had close ties with the research group of the RCGP. Again with advice from Robin Pinsent, I met several G.P.'s who had shown an interest in research and were becoming involved in it.

In Stockholm, an office with beautiful Scandinavian furniture had a long set of shelves behind the doctor's desk, for easy access to the large number of forms needed (exceeding even the paperwork required in British Columbia at the time). There was a mix of public and private medicine. The medical building had a private surgery suite with post-operative care and beds. Patients could have operations done privately 'tomorrow', rather than months later in the public system, but the range was restricted to the less complicated cases. At Goteberg, <u>Dr. Nels Blume</u> was among the first in Sweden to show an interest in research. The visit was memorable partly because he and his wife took us to the Liseborg Pleasure Gardens, where we adults ate a mountain of shrimp while their daughter took charge of our three children and gave them a good time.

In Denmark, we visited the small town of Ortved, near Ringstad. <u>Dr. Axel Bentzen</u> had his practice office in his home. His special interest was in body language, which gave clues about personality and problems of the patients. He loaned us his car for a short spin around the countryside. The natives were unusually friendly as they waved to us when we passed by, then we realized that his red sports car was easily recognizable. At lunch, our children quickly learned the meaning of 'skol', which gave them refills of their cokes.

For reasons forgotten, we missed contact with Dr. Chris van Deen in Groningen and Dr. Huygen in Utrecht. Both were active in the Netherlands College of General Practice which later published an annual booklet, *'Continuous Morbidity Registration'*, with recording by about fifty practitioners in Sentinel Stations, similar to the Epidemic Observation Unit of Dr. Ian Watson, to show the incidence of a selected number of conditions.

One of the lessons learned was to be very careful with notes and other papers gathered along the way. For the time in Europe and some of the time in the U.K., the notes which were to be sent to Victoria, B.C., Canada managed to get lost, after being misdirected to Victoria, Australia. This disaster was mitigated to some extent by the superb notes which Molly kept and organized, and our collective memory of some details.

Touchdown in Israel

After our time in Britain and Europe, Molly returned to Victoria in time for the children to start the school year. She found a reliable sitter, so that she could join me in mid-October in Sydney, Australia.

Travelling alone en route to Australia, on a non-medical stop in Jerusalem, by luck I met another Nuffield Fellow who was also staying at the YMCA - Dr. Michael Hutchinson from Worcester, who was in the public health program. Through him, I met Dr. Jack and June Medalie and Dr. Amos Arnon, working in very different settings and producing useful studies important to family medicine.

Dr. Medalie in Jerusalem had developed the Family Care Research Unit at Kiryat Hovel. There was a relatively small patient list, to allow time for research in family patterns of morbidity. He was conducting a major study of potential causes of coronary disease, involving 10,000 men and a large number of general practitioners. Later, as Professor of Family Medicine at the Case Western Reserve University in Cleveland, Ohio, he was active in promoting research in North America. He was a popular contributor to Canadian meetings, at NAPCRG and at WONCA. He wrote a useful textbook *'Family Medicine, Principles and Applications'* (Medalie, J., 1978).

A new Department of Medical Ecology (the first in the world) was at the Hadassah Medical School in Jerusalem. Dr. Michael Davies dealt with social and occupational factors which might contribute to the patterns of disease. He also was studying family patterns of disease.

Dr. Arnon practised in the small community of Nehora, about seventy-five miles south of Jerusalem (the longest taxi ride I have ever taken, but worth it). His office was in a central village, ringed by six smaller villages, each about two miles away. Each small village had a nurse who was the first contact for patients. Those who needed to see the doctor were transported by a daily bus service. This sytem was a good example of the use of nurses who could take care of many of the problems, and made it feasible for Dr. Arnon to emphasize preventive care, with about half his contacts devoted to immunization and other preventive measures. He developed a system of recording diagnoses and followup of patients and families, which he published in a book 'My Practice in my Pocket' (Arnon, A., 1978) which makes it relatively simple for any general practitioner to keep an accurate record of individual and family problems. He preferred to treat patients at home, rather than in the hospital which was in Beersheba. On one occasion when he was away, the hospital admission rate by his locum tenens was about double his usual rate. Later, he became the Professor of Family Medicine at Charleston, South Carolina.

Spring in Australia

Landing at Perth in the middle of the night during a thunderstorm was an impressive introduction to Australia, followed by a beautiful day of sunshine. The end of September was a good time to arrive, and the next six weeks were busy with visits to many of the general practitioners who were involved with research.

The activity of the thunderstorm typified the great activity in research across the country, much of it initiated and supported by the Australian College of General Practitioners at the state or national level. Various individual and group studies had been done or were in progress, some described in the *Annals of General Practice.* Many more were listed in a bibliography (Research Digest, 1968) which included studies over a ten-year period.

The Western Australia Chapter of the College had an active research committee. An evaluation of 850 obstetrical cases in his own practice was done by Dr. John Bamford in Perth. A similar study of his own obstetrical care was done by Dr. Kevin Cullen of Busselton, south of Perth, with a followup study showing improvement in outcomes after improved obstetrical care (Cullen, K.J., 1953). Dr. Cullen later did a study of behaviour disorders in children, involving 1,000 families (Cullen, K.J., 1965) as an M.D. thesis.

Dr. Bamford also had done a double-blind study of Herpes Zoster. He described the techniques involved (Bamford, J.A.C., 1963) and the problems in a study of a relatively uncommon disease.

In Adelaide, South Australia, a two-year survey of general practice had been done by Dr. Cliff Jungfer, a senior member of the Australian College. It was similar to the well-known surveys by Clute in Canada and Osler Peterson in the U.S.A., but different because he was an experienced general practitioner. Those visited were selected as representative, and data were analyzed on 108 physicians to describe the organization, scope and quality of performance (Jungfer, C., 1965). His tour was intended to be an educational outreach, in which he might offer advice as he observed a practitioner at work and later had time to discuss his observations. He was sometimes able to advise about practice methods or the need for further training.

A virus-spotting service had been started by Dr. Sorby Adams, also in Adelaide, for early recognition and reporting of virus infections. This was similar to the Virus Watch developed later by the Canadian College for recording the occurrence of influenza across Canada, since 1976. A similar project was being developed in Sydney by Dr. Alan Chancellor.

In Melbourne, Victoria, Dr. Ian Rowe was involved in various studies. He had led a group study of postpartum hemorrhage, including 2,796 cases and 68 members of the Australian College (Rowe, I.L., 1962) Also, he was an early and consistent contributor to research activity in Australia, including the National Morbidity Survey, and to WONCA.

Also in Melbourne, Dr. Alex McQueen Thomson had a major interest in preventive medicine, which involved an especially careful search for early signs of cancer at routine examination. Of 53 cases with no presenting symptoms, a five-year survival rate was seen in 100% of cases, compared with an overall rate of 65-70% in all cases of cancer. He also had a two-step test box for early detection of coronary insufficiency.

Many of the general practitioners contributing to the major studies were also doing individual studies, often in solo practice. In Traralgon, southeast of Melbourne, Dr. Charles Bridges-Webb conducted a survey of anesthetics given in general practice in the state of Victoria (Bridges-Webb, C., 1967), after a study in his own practice (Bridges-Webb, C., 1963). He had also done a three-year study of respiratory infections, which can be studied best in general practice (Bridges-Webb, C., 1964). He maintained an E Book for six consecutive years for an M.D. thesis at Monash University. After fifteen years in Traralgon, he moved to Sydney when appointed to the Chair of Community Medicine at the University of Sydney.

In Sydney, New South Wales (NSW), the headquarters of the Australian College of General Practice was in Bligh House (memories of Mutiny on the Bounty) where we were privileged to stay. Molly rejoined me there for the remaining two months of the Nuffield tour. I had promised her a trip to the Great Barrier Reef – as a biologist, she remembers this as the treat of a lifetime.

One of the first to record morbidity in his practice was Dr. John Radford of Sydney, chairman of the Research Committee of Council from 1958-1966. He recorded his experience for one year with the E Book (Radford, J.G., 1963 and 1964).

A large National Morbidity Survey had been done by the ACGP between February 1, 1962, and January 31, 1963. Assistance was provided by the Commonwealth Health Department and the Bureau of Census and Statistics. After three pilot surveys, the final version of an encounter card was completed for each patient visit in the year, by 85 family doctors recording 306,257 contacts (Breinl, W., 1964). The research committee produced a series of papers, with members taking sections of the data to write for publication when ready, rather than wait for one large report.

A similar survey was organized by Dr. Neville Andersen in Sydney, NSW, (Andersen, N.A., 1968). It involved a large number of general practitioners from a random sample. His study, in addition to the usual details of diagnosis, age and sex included an assessment of the extent of counselling and guidance, referrals to specialists, and work done in hospital. In 1976 he succeeded me as chairman of the research committee of WONCA.

In the village of Tea Gardens, NSW, Dr. Hanns Pacy did studies relevant to his area, near a beautiful beach extending 26 miles. His account of holiday hazards included insects, stingrays and sharks (Pacy, H., 1961) – which we heard about *after* we had jumped into the surf. He also contributed to the emergency care on a dangerous stretch of the main highway in a remote area (Pacy, H., 1967). He could reach the scene of an accident more quickly than the ambulance from the city of Newcastle. He had equipment in his car for first aid and resuscitation, to give victims a greater chance of survival.

Heading north to Queensland, in Brisbane we renewed acquaintance with Ben and Joyce Adsett, who had stayed with us a year earlier during Ben's Nuffield tour. Through them, we arranged for our memorable trip to the Great Barrier Reef. In Brisbane, Dr. Gordon Wright had conducted the Queensland Asthma Survey, to show the connection between weather and asthma. He found an increase of asthma in the autumn, not explained by pollen or spore counts but coinciding with inversion layers (Wright, G.L.T., 1964).

Finale in New Zealand

New Zealand was not so advanced in research as Australia. A stretched-out country with a smaller population, mostly in four cities, it was difficult and expensive to arrange national meetings. However, there was a growing interest in research; it seemed more on a faculty or individual level than national. As in the U.K., Europe and Australia we were guided by suggestions of Robin Pinsent, who had been an advisor to the New Zealand College of General Practitioners.

The first chairman of the research committee, Dr. E.J. Marshall, was a pioneer in the use of cervical smears, and in morbidity recording (Marshall, E.J., 1963). Morbidity recording in New Zealand was mainly in the E Book, of which there were about fifty. In 1965 there was no centralized collection of data.

One addition to the E Book was developed by Dr. C. Morrison, of Dunedin, who included illness which was not attended by the doctor. This was to give some way of relating minor illness to later major illness. Dr. Morrison also had an interest for over fifteen years in the use of chloroquin in subacute or chronic inflammatory conditions (Morrison, C.S., 1963).

A simple and encouraging survey of glycosuria was done in his practice by Dr. Geoff Gordon, in Kaikoura (north of Christchurch). He found only two new cases of diabetes; his regular routine seemed to be effective in detecting most cases. This type of result should be published, to counteract the impression sometimes given that there is a large reservoir of undetected disease.

Dr. Ashley Aitkin, in Oamaru on the South Island, had devised a summary card for recording significant details from patient contacts and basic details about past and family history. This was useful when adapted to our practice in Victoria, especially for thick files from which we could remove excess paper such as laboratory and x-ray reports.

In Wellington, on the southern edge of the North Island, it had been noted that hemoglobin levels in infants were low. A group study was underway, organized by Dr. Penry Putnam, to obtain data about hemoglobin levels in normal infants.

In Auckland, Dr. Deryck Gallagher was chairman of the national research committee. He had led a group study of acute urinary tract infections, showing that only 59% of those with symptoms had infections, of which 60% were from E. coli and 30% from Staphylococcus (Gallagher, D.J., 1965).

A way of keeping track of recurring problems was used by Dr. Rae West of Waiuku, a coastal town south of Auckland. For a specific complaint, such as headache, joint pain, hypertension or indigestion, a form was used to record pertinent details to compare with later progress. He had also developed a method of recording data during pregnancy to predict the date of delivery (West, S.R., 1965).

Among various studies in the planning stage was a survey of hospital admissions in Christchurch, to follow the progress of the patient after referral to specialist treatment. As hospitals in New Zealand were almost completely closed to general practitioners, there was a question whether the G.P. could contribute well to the care of his own patients.

WONCA

WONCA = World Organization of National Colleges and Academies of General Practitioners/Family Physicians and Allied Academic Institutions.

After the 1964 meeting in Montreal, sessions were held every two years in various parts of the world. Each session provided opportunities for general practitioners to meet informally and to give talks about their areas of interest. There was special interest in education and research, but any topic relevant to general practice could be submitted. The classification committee worked hard to produce the first version of the ICHPPC (International Classification of Health Problems in Primary Care). With Dr. Robert Westbury of Calgary, Alberta, as chairman, ICHPPC expanded on the Canuck Classification which he had developed with Dr. Michael Tarrant, also of Calgary. It became widely accepted as the best way to produce results which could be compared between countries. In 2001 it is still in use in a second edition, revised.

WONCA had a permanent base in Melbourne for administration, with Dr. David Game as director. The president for each term was elected from the country which was to be host for the next session. WONCA grew quickly, as more countries joined, and it has been a major factor in the recognition of general practice as an important asset in countries where it had not been well-organized previously.

Retrospective

In reviewing the names mentioned above, I am reminded that there were many more curious individuals who were working alone or in a group project, to contribute to the body of knowledge needed to show what general practice was and to identify areas which could be improved.

I am also reminded of the generous hospitality which we received along the way. Inexperienced in travel, I made arrangements which I would not make today. I am grateful for the advice I received about people and places to visit. All the contacts made confirmed for me that research in general practice was alive and well, and impressed me with the talent of so many family doctors in private practice. The exposure to their ideas and accomplishments was a stimulus to undertake more research on my own, and to contribute to the development of research in Canada. Canada had a long way to go.

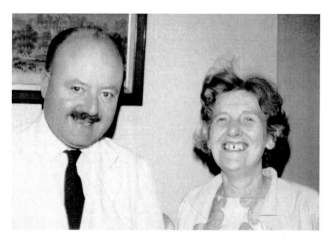

Dr. Robin and Ruth Pinsent, 1965

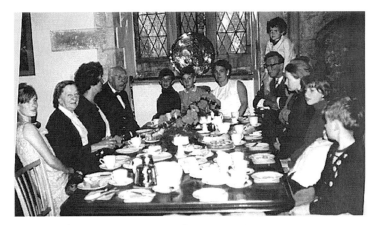

The Bill Fosters and the Bill Falks
at high tea in Bolton Castle, Aysgarth,
with Dr. and Mrs. Bill Pickles, 1965

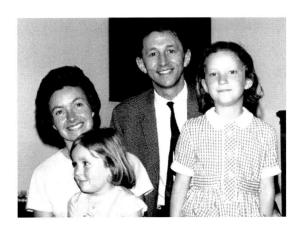

Dr. Ian and Dr. Betty McWhinney
with Heather and Julie
Stratford-upon-Avon, 1965

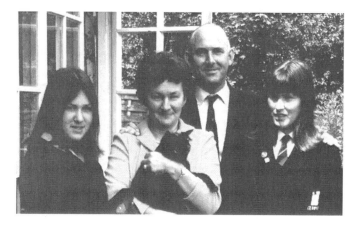

Dr. W.O. and Sheila Williams, Diana and Ann, Swansea, 1965

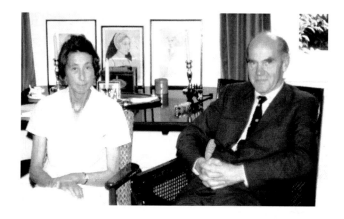

Dr. Edgar
and Eleanor
Hope-Simpson,
In Cirencester,
1965

Molly
and our three
in the Alps,
1965

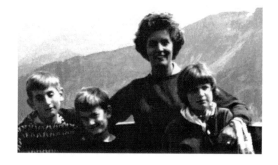

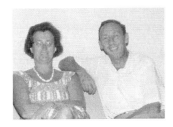

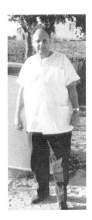

Dr. Jack and June Medalie
Jerusalem, 1965

Dr. Amos Arnon
Nehora , 1965

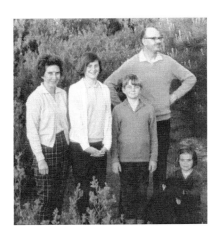

Dr. Ian and Patricia Rowe
Melbourne, 1965, with
Susan, Christopher and Julie

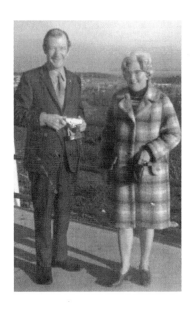

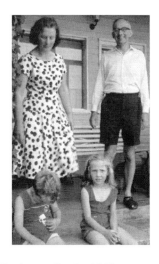

In Australia in 1965 ...
(top left) Dr. Neville and Pat
Andersen, Sydney
(above) Dr.Hanns and Marlene
Pacy, John and Marlene,
Tea Gardens, NSW

(bottom left) Dr. Clifford
Jungfer, Adelaide
(below) Dr. Ben and Joyce
Adsett, Brisbane

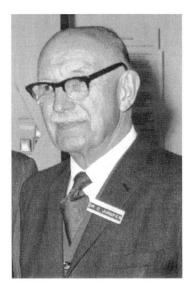

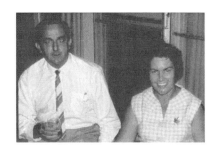

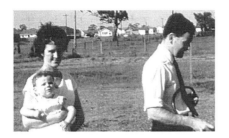

Dr. Charles and Anne Bridges-Webb
with Andrew, Traralgon, Victoria,
Australia, 1965

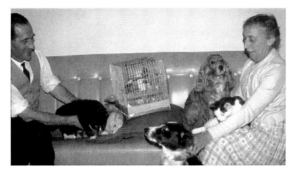

Dr. John and Molly Radford, Sydney,
with Robbie, Lisa, Tiddles, Frisky, Mandy
and (in the cage) Gussy, 1965

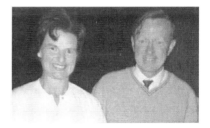

Dr. Rae and Lilian West
Waiuku, New Zealand, 1965

23

Chapter 2

Early Activity in Canada

A family physician might not consider doing research work partly because the very word 'research' carries with it the concept of high-powered institutions and laboratories. Again, with no training in or motivation to do research he would find enough satisfaction in general practice itself, for it offered a variety of interest and responsibility. The most common pattern of practice in Canada, even in cities, included hospital care, surgery, obstetrics and house calls. Even so, curiosity might lead him to wonder about some aspect of his practice. He would set out to find answers to his questions, organize his findings to learn something of interest to himself, and sometimes come up with original observations that could be of value to others – if tested and published.

This type of work, which was truly research, was termed 'Organized Curiosity' by Dr. Teviot Eimerl (Eimerl, T.S., 1960). It might be called 'evaluation', or simply 'study'.

Interesting studies have been done about general practice by general practitioners and non-general practitioners as well, the latter usually in the realm of public health or sociology. In this book, the main objective is to show what general practitioners have been inspired to do, often with help from experts but basically following up on their own curiosity.

Early studies in Canada

In Canada there are early examples of research done by general practitioners and published in journals not listed in the Index Medicus, or not published at all.

An example of the instinct to describe the work of the general practitioner was found recently by Dr. David

25

Shephard (Shephard, D.A.E., 1998). The medical manuscripts of Dr. John Mackieson of Charlottetown, P.E.I., in the 1890's, included two sets of case records, a synopsis of the medical conditions that were common in his practice, and a formulary of the drugs he used. This previously unpublished body of work could well have been typical of many other practitioners who kept track of their patients and their diagnoses.

Dr. W.C. Gibson, medical historian at the University of British Columbia, told of the work of Dr. W.D. Keith in the isolated Pemberton Valley of British Columbia. Endemic goitre was threatening the life and health of the population and the cattle. Dr. Keith investigated the situation and corresponded with a Dr. Marine in the U.S.A., to learn about the use of iodine in treatment. When he used it in Pemberton, there were dramatic improvements (Gibson, W.C., 1978).

The example cited above, of Dr. Mackieson's work, was found in browsing through the Canadian Medical Association Journal. There are probably many other records which might be discovered by a thorough search of the literature or of personal papers.

Studies in the 1950s

In the town of Duncan, B.C., on Vancouver Island, Dr. Peter Postuk kept a record of patient encounters in his group practice for a period of eight years from 1956. As there were no precedents nor good sources of advice readily available at the time, he used the classification of diseases in the Merck Manual, a popular handbook then in use for general practice. It was a practical guide, but not compatible with the International Classification of Diseases (I.C.D.), which was the standard. Eventually, in 1963, with the help of Dr. Cortland Mackenzie at the University of British Columbia, he was able to translate his findings for 1961 and 1962 into the approved classification, which was then accepted for publication (Postuk, P.D., 1969). He showed comparisons with the total population of patients and doctors in the district, to demonstrate that the study practice was representative of the area. The detailed list of conditions recorded was similar to other studies from general practice. One area of special interest was the category of "Neuropsychiatric and Psychosomatic", with a primary diagnosis made in only 3% of the total diagnoses. As in my own records, the number of psychiatric diagnoses was relatively small unless it included the anxiety component of any illness or injury. Postuk stressed the need for a classification of diseases appropriate for general practice in Canada.

With the easy availability of cervical cytology in B.C., Dr. Robert Lane, of Chilliwack, kept a record of papanicolau smears for six full years, 1958-1963 (Lane, R.F., 1965). Of 723 patients, 300 were tested because of symptoms. A total of 1,120 smears were done; 465 patients had only one test. Two invasive cancers were found, and thirteen carcinomas-in-situ. Of the fifteen patients who tested positive, only one showed normal cells on the first examination, and she was found to have abnormal cells on one-year followup.

In Creston, a town in the Kootenay region of British Columbia, Dr.Vern Murray kept a careful record of 1,618 deliveries over 23 years, reported in 1959 (Murray, J.V., 1959). He noted a trend to fewer long and difficult labours, and better judgement in recognition and treatment of complications. Labour was normal in 86% of deliveries.

Studies in the 1960s

During this decade, the central research committee of the College was trying to stimulate the membership to do research, and feeling frustrated by the lack of response. In fact, much activity was going on by a number of general practitioners who were curious about some aspect of their work. Many were in the smaller centres, but there were also many in the cities. The following list shows some of the topics that caught their imaginations. There has never been a shortage of topics to study, only the shortage of time and commitment to do the work.

Hypertension

One of the most popular topics for study has been high blood pressure. It is attractive because of the ease of measurement and the frequency, so that even in a solo practice there would be enough cases to be a respectable cohort. It is measurable by equipment normally found in all offices. In reading reports on hypertension studies, it is appropriate to look for a description of the conditions for taking the readings, as the Hopkinsons have done.

The Hopkinsons, a husband and wife team in Lion's Head, Ontario, conducted a study of uncomplicated hypertension, selecting fifty patients from office encounters, with pressures over 200/90 or with diastolic pressure over 100, with the patient seated and reassured. In 1961, they reported (Hopkinson, M.A. and N.E.J., 1961) that on treatment with a combination of hydrochlorothiazide 50mg, butabarbital 30 mg, and reserpine 0.5 mg. over a twelve-week period, the average drop in diastolic pressure was 9.3 mm and in systolic pressure was 54.3. Minor side-effects were seen in 22%, and drug failures in 6%.

Another study in hypertension was conducted at the McMaster Medical Centre over thirteen years, starting in 1965. Vince Rudnick et al described an organized effort to detect and treat hypertension, and to document follow-up and outcomes. They showed a decrease in mortality from strokes and heart failure with good control of hypertension (Rudnick, K.V., 1979). Measurement of blood pressure during routine office visits was emphasized, so that the level of recording rose from 41% at the beginning to 98% at the end of the study. The number of new hypertensive patients was high in the first five years, dropping to a low yield towards the end.

Heart disease

In the town of High Prairie, Alberta, Dr. Philip Rutter

began a ten-year study of myocardial infarction, from January 1, 1963 to December 31, 1972. Of 72 cases, 66 were confirmed by ECG, transaminase, and/or autopsy; 65 patients were involved, six having two or three incidents. Only ten cases were seen in the native population, which made up about half the practice population. Dr. Rutter thought that the prognosis for survival was worse than in the city (Rutter, P., 1974).

A five-year study of coronary disease started on January 1, 1968 by Dr. Douglas P. Black in Baie Verte, Newfoundland. He aimed to determine the most appropriate type of facility for treatment of myocardial infarction in his rural community, where there was a low incidence and a low death rate in infarctions. He concluded that there was no need in his community for a coronary care unit. Smaller areas should look carefully at their own need before they commit the large cost to establish a coronary care unit.

The content of practice

Dr. Peter Postuk followed the afore-mentioned long-term study in his practice (in the 1950's) with a short-term study in 1964 involving 54 general practitioners in British Columbia (Postuk, P.D.,1972). They recorded details of patient contacts, using a list of 43 diagnostic categories adapted from the International Classification of Diseases. Diagnoses, place of contact, and time spent were recorded for periods varying from one day to 72 days. The overall average number of contacts per day was about 30. In urban practices 65.9% were seen in the office and 22.1% in the hospital. In rural practices 53.8% were seen in the office and 35.8% in hospital. "Rurban" practices were in between, with 60.5% and 29.3 %.

A study of morbidity in six family practices in Newfoundland was conducted by Dr. John Ross, of St. John's, financed by a National Health Grant (Ross, J., 1972). Over a period from January 1966 to May 1967, morbidity was recorded in the E Book, using the classification of the Royal College of General Practitioners in Britain (RCGP), for inpatient and outpatient contacts. In six rural practices, including five which were based on cottage hospitals, all illness episodes were recorded, as well as other items of service. Variations between practices seemed to correlate with the presence of cottage hospitals. Ross suggested that the data could be useful in planning health care, and that much of the preventable illness seemed due to disadvantageous social forces.

This early study served as a basis of comparison with other practices in Canada, as well as in other countries (Ross, J., 1972). In 1969, a transatlantic morbidity study was reported by the Newfoundland Chapter of the College of Family Physicians of Canada and the Research Unit of the Royal College of General Practitioners. It compared morbidity of immigrants to Newfoundland with morbidity of their families or former neighbours in Devon or in Ireland, in groups chosen according to the names of patients (Transatlantic, 1969).

A different approach was used by MacFarlane and O'Connell, who extracted data from records on a 23% random sample of family medicine patients in the McMaster University Clinic in Hamilton, Ontario. Over a 12-month period, October 1967 to November 1968, they recorded symptoms and diagnoses (MacFarlane, A.H., 1969). They noted a high frequency of pain, respiratory problems (particularly infection), emotional problems, and degenerative problems (particularly obesity and cardiovascular).

A landmark study, "The Work of a Group of Doctors in Saskatchewan", was carried out in the Saskatoon Community Clinic in 1964, describing the twelve-month experience of the six general practitioners, a surgeon, and a psychiatrist. The study was designed and written by Dr. Sam Wolfe and Dr. Robin Badgely, and the daily organization was maintained by Dr. John Garson. In addition to the comprehensive summary of the work of the doctors, and some comparison with other studies, there is a review of the literature with many useful references. (Wolfe, S. et al, 1968). This study was included in the

Milbank Memorial Fund Quarterly (MMFQ) of January, 1968. A much more detailed study was published in a special edition of the MMFQ about the general practitioner (Wolfe, S. et al, 1972).

Some of the studies of family/general practice were conducted by non-general practitioners. A study of doctor/patient contacts in family practice was done by a group in the Department of Preventive Medicine at Queens University, that included Dr. Peter Smith as the family physician (Steele, R. et al, 1968). Twelve family physicians were asked to record patient contacts for seven days, each day of the week being chosen once during a seven-week period. Age-groups, diagnoses, costs, and severity of illness were reported in this exploratory study. This example shows the realization by other disciplines of the importance of general practice.

Workload

Work in a multispecialty group in Toronto was recorded for a six month period in 1968 by Dr. A. Shardt (Shardt, A., 1969). In the first part of the study he dealt with patterns of practice. The group included nine general practitioners, four of whom were partners and five were salaried assistants, plus a surgeon and an internist. Laboratory and X-ray services were provided by a part-time radiologist and a pathologist. Differences between the partners and assistants were seen in the number of office visits, house calls and charges. Physician contacts were 92% in the office, and 2.5% by house calls, most of which were done by the salaried assistants. Apart from surgery and obstetrics, there were only 33 hospital visits.

The emergency department

While director of the General Practice Service in the Emergency Department of the Vancouver General Hospital, Dr. John Zack conducted a six-month study of the patients seen there. As reported in 1967 (Zack, J.J., 1967), he found that 61% of patients were self-referred, and of those about 20% were "true emergencies". Those referred by physicians were judged to be true emergencies in 86% of patients requiring treatment or admission.

A similar study was done by <u>Dr. Teglas</u> in Toronto (Teglas, A.L., 1969) involving 3,249 patients seen by their attending family practitioners. He found that 70% of cases were rated as minor medical or surgical problems, 11.1% were intermediate-major, and 19.9% were major (of which 9.0% were surgical and 9.9% medical). Even in those days there was a problem of disposal of patients because of a lack of doctors, pressure on diagnostic facilities, and shortage of hospital beds.

<u>Dr. C.M. Baars</u> compiled data on patients visiting the emergency department of Riverside Hospital in Ottawa, for one week in May, 1968. Questionnaires were completed by 386 patients, and by 383 staff members. Two followup questionnaires were completed by 105 patients (27%). Even then, the ratio of non-urgent to urgent cases was two-to-one. X-rays were done on 14%, lab tests on 3%, 14% received prescriptions, and 43% had injections or minor surgery. Three percent were admitted to hospital. The follow-up by regular physicians was about 40% (Baars, C.M., 1969).

Infectious disease

While a polio epidemic was occurring in Montreal and Quebec City, a different epidemic was underway in Donnacona, Quebec. Antibody studies showed the presence of Coxsackie B5 virus in 37 cases, as reported by College member <u>Dr. Rosaire Cauchon</u> in 1960 (Cauchon R., 1960). The clinical syndrome was seen in 250 cases, with mild to severe symptoms. Treatment with injections of vitamins P and C seemed to improve the symptoms and outcome.

One of the few females to publish a research study was <u>Dr. Yvonne de Buda</u>, who recorded a small but significant series of ten cases of asymptomatic proteinuria detected on routine testing. After investigation, final diagnoses were:: glomerulonephritis (2); pyelonephritis (3) (including one with renal calculus and urethral stricture; renal tuberculosis in one; multiple myeloma in one); and three undetermined, two of which were considered to be orthostatic albuminuria (de Buda.Y., 1967).

Another study of urinary tract infections was done by Drs. Donald Brown and Kwang Yang, doing routine urinalysis on 690 children aged up to fifteen, during twelve months from June 1, 1967 (Brown, D., 1972). Urinary tract infection was diagnosed in 102 (14.8%), half of whom had fever when first seen. Only eight were symptomless, and thirty presented with respiratory infection. The authors emphasized the need to identify, treat and follow episodes of infection, to avoid chronic infection in later life.

Dr. Walter Rosser was involved in a study, with Dr. J.G. Simms, of farmer's lung in urbanites (Simms, J.G., 1970). On the basis of one identified case, tests were done on 37 members of a riding club in Kanata, Ontario. Of these, five were found to have antibodies to Thermopolyspora. The reported case was the only one requiring medical attention, but it was thought that workers in the stables, with much longer exposure, would be at risk.

Dr. Peter Heaton sent a questionnaire to a sample of family physicians in Ontario, asking about use of antibiotics in treatment of uncomplicated upper respiratory infections. The response of 67% (without follow-up) showed that 42% used antibiotics rarely, 43% about half the time, and 15% usually. They also listed the indications for which they would use antibiotics in cases with complications. Patient pressure was often a problem (Heaton, P., 1973).

Economics

In a conference on the Costs and Organization of Medical Care, held in Saskatoon in 1969, results of two research projects by general practitioners in the Saskatoon Community Clinic were presented. Dr. John Bury, in a study of the prescribing rates and costs of drugs, found that patients with a plan for paying for prescriptions filled almost twice as many of the prescriptions written as those without a plan. He suggested that the use of a formulary of approved drugs would lower the cost of drugs, so that otherwise unfilled prescriptions might be affordable (Bury, J.D., 1969).

Dr. John Garson reported on a study of "Checkups - Useful or Useless". In considering the many pros and cons, he was firmly in favour of the check-up or screening program, provided that it is relevant and makes use of modern technology for data storage and retrieval, and also modern equipment for multiphasic screening. He advocated that appropriate use of doctors, nurses, clerks, and other personnel would be necessary in a multidisciplinary approach to health education (Garson, J.Z., 1969).

Mental health

Dr. Jim Collyer, in London, Ontario, had a special interest in psychiatric care, shown in his study in Psychiatric Care in General Practice (Collyer, J.A., 1968). With the advice of Dr. Harding Leriche, he evaluated his findings according to defined criteria. Of the 53 patients in the study, 9 were considered to have poor response to the average of six hours of therapy, 3 were chronic, 10 were improved and 31 had excellent results.

Collyer also did a five-month study of time spent with patients, including those needing psychotherapy. He found that the average time per consultation was 14.8 minutes, with 21.1 minutes per psychotherapy visit and 9.8 minutes for other visits (Collyer, J.A., 1969a). He followed this study with a similar approach involving eight other family doctors, who recorded experience with 69 patients with psychosomatic symptoms. Although eight patients were referred to a psychiatrist or a clinic, five were returned for followup and the family doctors treated 92% of the sample. In followup, 60% were relieved or normal, 26% improved but chronic, and 13% no better. However, as Collyer concluded, the method was too complicated to be practical. One surprising response from physicians was that "two minutes was too long to expect a man in practice to take in filling out forms, particularly for more than one or two patients per month" (Collyer, J.A., 1969b).

Dr. D.G. Workman did a six-month study of the effect

of psychotropic drugs on prison inmates, to assess acts of aggression. He found that those on antianxiety agents (especially diazepam) had 3.6 times more incidents of aggression than those not on medication. He noted that the group in prison had a highly aggressive history, but that similar tendencies might be a problem with aggressive patients on psychotropic drugs who are not in prison (Workman, D.G., 1975).

In a study of mental health care for the Alberta Chapter of The College, Dr. Howard Gretton in Calgary, Alberta, received responses from 80 members. Half were in solo practice, half in groups. Half were in cities of over 50,000. Gretton stressed the point that family physicians are interested in total patient care and regard mental health as part of total health. The average respondent had a yearly case-load of eighty patients who required counselling and interviewing. One patient a month was referred to a psychiatrist, one every three months to an Alberta Psychiatric Hospital and less than one a month to a social agency. The majority reported inadequate information from the hospital on discharge of their patients. Only six respondents reported lack of interest when dealing with psychiatric problems (Gretton, A. H., 1968).

At the Community Clinic in Regina, Saskatchewan, income from clinical work was used to support the salary of a psychiatric social worker, Len Ghan. He and Dr. David Road published a monograph with results of their analysis of interactions between the psychotherapist, doctors, and patients over two years, 1966-68 (Ghan, L., 1970).

A study of family therapy was done at the McMaster University Clinic, with a matched control group (Comley, A., 1973). In the study group, the number of visits per year for all conditions decreased by 50% in the year after family therapy.

Manpower

Morgan and Mansfield in 1968 studied the geographic distribution and availability of physicians in Vancouver, B.C. (Morgan, R.W, 1969). They used the telephone book as a guide to those who were available. This method I have found to be the most useful and closest to the real number of general practitioners available to the public, when compared with official lists from the College of Physicians and Surgeons and the Medicare system. Morgan found that in the city, as in the province, there was not an even distribution, as there was a heavier concentration of physicians near the major hospitals. Only 19% of physicians would not take new patients. Of general practitioners, 35% would not take new patients, with the most recent graduates more willing to accept them (78%).

In 1967, Dr. Fred Fallis began a study of general practice manpower in Metropolitan Toronto as a first step towards a better understanding of basic problems and trends in the delivery of urgent and primary health care (Fallis, F., 1971). He found many inconsistencies in the existing lists. A mailed questionnaire to get more accurate information yielded 521 replies, of which only 451 were in active general practice. Telephone followup, personal enquiry, and word of mouth brought the total of practising general practitioners up to 690. Fallis's experience is similar to my own in assessing family practice manpower in Victoria and in British Columbia - it is necessary to have local knowledge in order to make accurate lists. The data were used to produce a register of Toronto general practitioners and details about their location, training, languages spoken, type of practice and availability.

In 1969 a program was established to place physicians in areas of Ontario deemed to be underserviced (Bass, M. and Copeman, W.J., 1975a). From then to 1973, 162 communities were designated as underserviced, and 196 physicians were placed. Modern facilities were built by seventy-five communities to attract physicians. Some students who had received bursaries for going to a designated practice area returned after graduation (53% of the first group) but the long-term service was not yet known.

Services

Dr. Shardt published two other articles based on the study of the practice from 1960 to 1969. Even then, there was a shortage of manpower in general practice. In the last three years of the study his group of five family physicians delivered 11.8 % of maternity patients, compared with 12% for the other 43 family physicians on staff of the Toronto General Hospital. The other 76% were delivered by obstetricians. When considering all the other demands on time, he concluded that it might be better to delegate some part of obstetrical care to properly-trained and supervised nurses, nurse-midwives, and allied health personnel (Shardt, A., 1970).

Potpourri

In Red Deer, Alberta, a double-blind study with random allocation of 50 patients was reported by Dr. Jack Staples. It showed that Halperidol had a potentiating effect on the action of meperidine, with good tranquilizing and anti-emetic action and no apparent side-effects (Staples, J.C., 1967).

In 1966, Dr. Michael Livingston in Richmond, B.C., began a one-year follow-up study of 60 patients whom he treated by spinal manipulation. Results were good or excellent in 45 patients, with over 50% improvement in another eight (Livingston, M., 1969). None was made worse. It was concluded that spinal manipulation was an effective method of treating the spinal syndromes. Livingston had long experience and training in manipulation. He emphasized the necessity for such training before using the methods on patients.

A screening program aimed at identifying hyperparathyroidism was reported by Dr. David Lawee of Toronto, Ontario. He included one thousand patients from

May 11, 1964, to July 22, 1965, with results of calcium and phosphorus tests (Lawee, D., 1970). One case of hyperparathyroidism (post-thyroidectomy) was identified, which might have been evident clinically.

Dr. Walter Rosser studied a small selected group of patients to assess their conformity with discharge instructions. They found that those who were given written instructions rather than oral, followed them more consistently. He felt that these findings should be followed with a larger study to identify their reasons for differences in compliance. (Rosser, W.W., 1971).

The primary health care role of the pharmacist was studied by Dr. Martin Bass in London, Ontario (Bass, M., 1975b). Problems were treated by non-prescription medication in 80%, 12% were referred for medical care, and 8% received reassurance and information.

*   *   *

Activity in research was increasing in the late 60s, according to the number of publications which appeared in the literature available to me. Some reports were published years after the project had been started or completed, notably the above-mentioned thirteen-year study by Rudnick, which began in 1964 and was published in 1979, and the studies by Postuk.

Studies in the 1970s

The first half of the decade saw an increase in the number of studies done and published. Research had a greater visibility than before, with regular newsletters in the Canadian Family Physician, and multiple provincial and national workshops supported by The College, to provide basic training in research methods relevant to family practice.

The content of practice

A comparison of rural and urban family practice in similar two-man practices involved 2,600 patients in Vancouver and 2,687 patients in Castlegar over the same two-week period (Bartel G.G., 1970). Although the variety of problems was similar in city and country, the rural doctors spent more time in hospital, especially with surgery and anesthetics. The city doctors saw more older patients, compared with more patients aged 0-16 years in the rural practice.

During 1974, Dr. Tony Valentine in Winnipeg, Manitoba, maintained records in the E Book for all his patient care (Valentine, A.S., 1975). He described the age and sex distribution of patients and of morbidity. In comparing his figures with those of Ross, in Newfoundland, the differences showed the need to have data from a variety of settings, in order to guide the teaching of family practice residents in realistic preparation for their entry into the field.

A study of family practice in the small rural community of Rainy River in Northwestern Ontario was conducted through the year 1975 by Dr. Tony Dixon (Dixon, A.S., 1976, a & b). This very complete survey was recorded in the E Book, using the Canuck Classification. Dixon defined the population at risk and recorded morbidity in terms of illness episodes, referral patterns, use of a small hospital, and differences in morbidity between Indian and non-Indian patients. Among the large amount of relevant detail reported, the absence of neoplasm in the Indian population was of interest and perhaps warrants study on a larger population.

Therapy

A double-blind study of the effectiveness of aspirin or indomethacin, compared with a placebo was done by Dr. Gerald Pawlowski (Pawlowski, G.J., 1971). He found that both of the non-steroidal anti-inflammatories were significantly more effective than placebo in relieving local tenderness and limitation of movement and that indomethacin also relieved pain on movement.

Four family physicians in Winnipeg performed cultures on 540 patients complaining of sore throat, during one year. They withheld treatment until results of the cultures were known, and made a clinical judgment of viral or strep throat. The initial clinical judgment was wrong almost as often as it was right. Only 10.1% of cultures were positive for Streptococcus Group A. Without cultures, 245 patients would have been treated, 190 unnecessarily, and 22 cases of strep throat would not have been treated. (Hart, W.J., 1976).

Nurse practitioners

A pilot project, with a family practice nurse as primary contact in small villages in the area of Baie Verte, Newfoundland, was organized to work with the group of salaried physicians at the medical centre in Baie Verte. This change was accepted by the communities involved, and appeared to improve the quality and availability of primary medical care (Black, D.P., 1976).

Classification of Problems

Drs. Michael Tarrant and Robert Westbury worked on the recording of problems in their group practice in Calgary, Alberta, and developed a classification appropriate for Canada, known as the Canuck Classification (Westbury R., 1969). This was useful as a step towards publication in 1975 of the The International Classification of Health Problems in Primary Care (ICHPPC) by The World Organization of National Colleges and Academies of General/Family Practice (WONCA). Dr. Westbury was chairman of the Classification Committee of WONCA, which included members from around the world, and which produced the practical list of diseases and problems which could be used in most family practice settings, to provide a basis of comparison of experience between countries.

Workload

A pilot study of the workload of family doctors in Alberta was conducted by Dr. Claude Labelle. Questionnaires were sent to 213 potential recorders of which 55 (24.4%) were returned (a few were not recorded properly, and were discarded). He found that about twenty patients per working day were seen in the office, eight patients in hospital, and less than one on house calls. When telephone calls were added, there were about 224 contacts per week, of which 182 were visits, averaging 60 hours per week (Labelle, C., 1973).

One of Bob Westbury's useful ideas in the field of communication was "The Electric Speaking Practice: a telephone workload study" (Westbury, R.C., 1974). Over two periods (eleven weeks from October 7 to December 21, 1970, and eight weeks from October 25 to December 17, 1971) he recorded the number of calls, their length, the day of the week, their purpose, and the other person involved. His detailed description of results rang true, and he showed that the service provided a saving in time for the patients and a saving of cost for the paying agencies, but brought no income to the practice.

Prevention

The 'check-up' has been advocated as necessary by various agencies which are not in the business of providing such a service, so that sometimes one might feel guilty for not having one every year. This concept was studied by Dr. J. Garson in the Saskatoon Community Clinic for six months in 1970. Patients completed a questionnaire before an examination and basic lab work. Compared with four doctors using the conventional history, the other four general practitioners in the group using the questionnaires provided more details of the patient's history, and an identified group for follow-up. Little extra time was taken by the doctor, in examining the patient and providing results (Garson, J.Z., et al 1972).

Abnormal results on nearly 10.5% of electrocardiograms led to further study to assess the number of significant findings. Patients aged forty or more had routine ECG's from January 2 to May 31, 1972. Of the 631 patients tested, significant abnormalities were seen in 60, insignificant abnormalities in 260, and normal results in 311. Under the age of 45, there were only three (3%) significant abnormalities, so that the routine use of ECG's in that group would not be likely to justify the expense. There was no report on how many of the findings were previously not known (Garson, J.Z., 1972a).

Quality of Care

A team at McMaster University took on the difficult topic of quality assessment in a one-year study of the Burlington practice. Three approaches were used: surveillance of the management of indicator conditions; evaluation of the clinical use of drugs; and the assessment of referral decisions. The findings could be useful for those studied, in determining the need for continuing education (Sibley, J.C., 1975).

Out of office calls

A study on the use and abuse of a hospital emergency department was done by Dr. S. Bain, with the help of an industrial engineer at the North York General Hospital in Toronto. In a 28-day period in July 1970, of the 80% of the sample of 3,622 patients who claimed to have a family doctor, only half phoned the family doctor before coming in. Some who were advised by the family doctor not to come in came in anyway. Both patient and physician agreed on 22 cases as being emergency or life-threatening. Patients rated 1,992 cases as non-urgent, while doctors rated 1,537 as non-urgent; they agreed on 1,020 cases, suggesting that 2,509 cases (69%) had been so judged by at least one responder. They suggested that there was a need for public education to encourage proper use of the emergency services (Bain, S., 1971).

A timely reminder that a weekend on call involves more than the emergency ward was provided by Dr. John Garson, who was on call for his group of eight general practitioners for 48 hours, starting at 8 a.m. on Saturday (Garson, J.Z., 1973). He described the wide range of conditions encountered, and the assessment of only two calls as frivolous. Ten patients were seen in the emergency ward, and fourteen at home.

In the group of ten family physicians in the Saskatoon Community Clinic, Dr. Phil Loftus found that in the year 1974 5.6% of the total of 51,000 services were provided in the home, emergency department, or nursing home (Loftus P., 1976). Only 2% were considered to be totally unwarranted, while 36% were urgent and 28% were 'fair enough'. The number of house calls almost doubled during the winter months. Figures were given for the clinic as a whole, because factors such as illness, research, and service to a small town in the country, caused variations in the time available for some members for doing house calls.

In Victoria, B.C., a study of waiting time in an emergency department was led by Dr. A.B. Allen in 1971 (Allen, A.B. et al, 1973). When extreme, life-threatening emergencies were included with serious but not life-threatening cases they amounted to 8% of the total after minor elective procedures (16.9%) were excluded. Minor emergencies then were classified in 67% and trivia (which could have been done in the physician's office the same or the next day) in 25%. The waiting times compared favorably with those in other studies. There was a small decrease when a full-time physician was available to supervise interns.

Weight problems

Dr. Jim Collyer did a retrospective study of 103 consecutive cases of obesity in his practice (Collyer, J.A., 1973). Using a variety of diets, hypnosis and medications, over an average of 23 weeks, he found an average weight loss of 10.5 pounds. He noted a high incidence of emotional problems, with 95% of patients, and considered that the obesity was often a result of these problems and that weight reduction was more successful when emotional problems were improved.

The Elderly

Family doctors are expected to be aware of social problems in their patients. During the year from April, 1973, a study was done on 92 elderly patients of the Saskatoon Community Clinic who required hospital care or treatment at home for major or acute illness. They found that 33% of patients had inadequate income, and that domiciliary physiotherapy and occupational therapy were needed. As a result of the study, a social worker was funded for the group practice by the provincial government (Garson, J.Z., & Wolfe, R.R.).

After using the E Book for one year, to record illness patterns in the office, Dr. Wayne Elford in Calgary, Alberta , focused on chronic illness. Nineteen conditions were selected, each with a section in the book. Each patient was listed on a separate page in the appropriate section or sections. This new approach was well-accepted by patients and the family practice nurse, and helped to provide better follow-up (Elford, R.W., 1975).

Potpourri

A record of 100 vasectomies was described by Dr. Collier (Collier, K.J., 1974) in a group of three family physicians in Portage La Prairie, Manitoba. Apart from one post-operative infection, morbidity was low and satisfaction high. In follow-up, patients volunteered many comments, which reinforced the conclusion that vasectomies are safe, easy to perform, economical and result in no psychological problems.

Manpower

Also in 1974, Dr. Martin Bass in London, Ontario, described the availability of family physicians, with all but one of 128 responding to his interviews, 122 in person and five by telephone and letter. The average family physician was 43.5 years old and in practice in London for 10.3 years. Workload per week averaged 128 patients in the office, 4.7 house calls, and 2.6 patients under his care in hospital plus 2.8 patients under referred care. New patients were accepted by 59 physicians, plus 46 who accepted patients on referral by a physician or another patient. Most tried to educate their patients on proper use of the emergency wards and specialists. It seemed that there were enough family physicians at that time, with a ratio of 1,800 patients to 1 (Bass, M., 1975).

Unpublications

Even the lists of family medicine literature do not contain all research done by family physicians, as there are certainly studies which have been completed but not published. For example, a survey of 320 general practitioners in B.C. was done in June, 1961, by Drs. Jim Fowler and Bill Falk to ask how many and what type of patient services they provided. This was done for the benefit of the provincial chapter of the College, to provide an estimate of the workload of the average G.P. It was useful at the time, but not submitted for publication (Fowler, J.A., 1962).

Responses showed an average work week in different areas varied from 59 to 66 hours, the shortest being in Vancouver and in areas with population under 5,000. The majority saw 16-25 patients per day in the office, with a few under ten and a few over 30. In hospital, the range was from 5 patients in Vancouver to 10 where population was less than 5,000. House calls were done in all areas, averaging two per day, the lowest being in Vancouver with 1.7. Even though this was a non-randomized sample of volunteer respondents, the results were considered to be credible in describing the range of work of the general practitioner.

Morbidity

In 1971, morbidity recording in the E Book was done in my group practice, along with four solo G.P.'s in B.C. – Dr. John Sumner and Dr. Brian Dixon-Warren in Maple Ridge (in separate practices), Dr. Brian Allen in Victoria, and Dr. Dennis Moore in Smithers. A research assistant was supported by a National Health Grant. The results were submitted for publication, but not accepted, although some of the material was useful in workshops (Falk, W.A., 1972).

In retrospect, it is probable that the report was not well enough written to be acceptable.

Even this small collection showed surprising differences in diagnoses between practices. The top ten diagnoses from each practice were widely variable. They included thirty-three items, with only two which were included in all practices (lacerations, etc, and tonsillitis). Psychiatric or psychoneurotic diagnoses were recorded in 9% (range 6 to 11% per physician) of patients in my group practice, which had an awareness of the importance of psychiatric problems, and an average of 7% (range 3 to 8%) in the four separate practices. If other diseases with a suspected psychoneurotic component were added, (asthma, hypothyroidism, hypertension, peptic ulcer, irritable bowel, eczema, or obesity) the totals ranged from 12.8% to 20.6% in my group, and 9.9% to 15.1% in the solo practices. These figures do not support the frequent statements by experts who have claimed that the majority of work in general practice is generated by neurotic problems. However, it must be considered that any disruption of usual health, such as a sprain, fracture, infection, or indigestion can cause some anxiety or depression until the problem is solved, so that a secondary diagnosis of anxiety or depression might be recorded.

Summation

There are many names mentioned which will be remembered by those who have had an interest in research. The number of mentions is not related to the number of works by individuals, but is a selection of those which show the range of topics and the variety of individuals.

Without judging the scientific quality of these earlier studies, the fact is that there were individual general practitioners who had enough interest to undertake projects and spend the time needed to complete them and submit them for publication. There were also some who did not go the final step toward publication but still learned something of interest to themselves and often provided material for presentation at meetings.

A rough count of the articles chosen to include in this chapter shows a majority by general practitioners in private practice, and relatively few in university settings. This is not surprising, as the first family medicine teaching programs did not begin in London and Calgary until 1966, and there was no medical school in Calgary at that stage. In the 1950s, the three studies were all in private practice. In the 1960s, about 80% of studies were in private practice. In the first five years of the 1970s, about 80% were in private practice. My impression is that now most projects are done or originated in the family practice units, rather than in private practice.

Chapter 3

The College Research Committees

In 1954 the newly-formed College of General Practice of Canada saw the need for education aimed at the work of general practitioners, starting with continuing education programs for those already in practice who wished to update their knowledge and skills. The concept of life-long learning was recognized as vital to the maintenance of competence in practice. The focus on postgraduate and undergraduate education came soon afterward at a time when it was the only organization of physicians on this continent to demand continuing education to maintain membership.

In contrast, the focus of the Royal College of General Practitioners in Britain (RCGP), founded in 1952, was on research from the beginning. There was a need to show what problems were faced by general practitioners. Methods were developed to describe the clinical content of practice, the workload, and the organized structure. It was logical that, in time, the Canadian college could provide some helpful advice when the British college became more involved in education for general practice. In return, the British college was a great source of inspiration and practical advice to the Canadian college and its members who became interested and involved in research.

Through the years there was an increasing amount of interchange of ideas and people between the Colleges in Canada and in other countries, especially those which have been described in Chapter 1.

The Research Committees

As with many committees, for economy it was usually best to select a chairman who would form a committee of interested members within a reasonable distance. The term would be about three years, to allow

49

enough time to become familiar with the problems and to establish policies. The first research committees were in Ontario, within reach of the College's headquarters.

The 1955 Research Committee - Toronto

The first annual report of the College, in 1956, described the first step towards a research program for Canadian general practitioners. The Board of Representatives of the College at its June, 1955, meeting directed that a committee on research be established. Dr. M.E.W. Gooderham of Don Mills, Ontario, was chairman. The committee's terms of reference were: "It shall explore the possibilities for research in general practice and encourage the study of research projects by family doctors in this country. It is to be the task of this committee to organize and coordinate a plan of medical research by the general practitioners of Canada."

The committee report stated that "we propose to make haste slowly, for we feel that we should not embark on too many projects at once". A form was included for anyone interested to register with the research committee, whether or not a member of the College.

While the research committtee was charged with developing an interest among members across Canada, there were plans for a large-scale survey of general practice by the College and the Department of Preventive Medicine of the University of Toronto. It had the support and active participation of the Canadian Medical Association and collaboration with the Rockefeller Foundation. Financial support was provided by the Canadian Life Insurance Officers Association and the Federal government. This survey was to be done by a well-qualified general practitioner or internist, who would visit a random sample of general practitioners and spend a few days with each to evaluate a list of factors:

- the educational background
- the quality of histories and records
- the quality of the physical examination
- laboratory work

- treatment
- working conditions
- educational programs
- differences between single, partnership, and group practices
- influence of prepaid medical and hospital care plans
- preventive medicine practised
- relationships with hospitals, specialists, public health officials and colleagues.

These activities are mentioned to show that there was an early acceptance by the College of the need for study of general practice, even though there had been little apparent activity in the field by general practitioners and the major survey planned was not connected with the research committee. The principle researcher was not even a general practitioner, but a pediatrician, Dr. K.F. Clute. His team of investigators included himself, an internist, and a "generalist" with postgraduate public health training. 'Canada' was represented by a sample of 86 practices in Ontario and Nova Scotia. The Ontario random sample of 56 Canadian-educated male physicians who had been listed as general practitioners two years earlier was reduced to 44 because of one death, one illness, five who were not general practitioners, and five who refused to participate. The results of the study, started in 1956, were published in 1963 in a book, "The General Practitioner" (Clute, K.F., 1963).

One of the earliest signs of subsequent activity was described in the Bulletin of the College of General Practice of Canada in November, 1957. It reported a study of Echo Virus type 9, a collaboration between general practitioners, medical health officers, and the University of Toronto School of Hygiene. It was recognized that "doctors in general practice are in a strategic position to assist in the investigation of [viral] illnesses, and their continued assistance is encouraged".

The 1958 Research Committee - London

In the third annual report of the College, in 1958, there is no mention of the research committee, except for naming the chairman, <u>Dr. E.S. Jeffrey</u> of London, Ontario. This report seemed to fulfill the previous stated policy of the committee to "make haste slowly". The executive director, Dr. Victor Johnston, reported that the first phase of the Survey of General Practice in Canada, by Dr. K. Clute, had been completed in Ontario.

Also in 1958, the Bulletin of the College of General Practice printed an invitation to Canadian general practitioners to participate with the Royal College of General Practitioners (RCGP) in a research program which was already well-established in Britain. The British College wished to establish a research network throughout the Commonwealth. It already had links with general practice organizations in Australia and New Zealand, and with medical faculties in Malaya and Kenya. Dr. Pinsent, chairman of the research committee of the RCGP, offered them access to the register of over 550 general practitioners and their research subjects. As he said, "the range of general practice is over the whole of medicine and most of surgery and obstetrics" ... "eighty percent of all episodes of illness which appear in the doctor's consulting room or the home also end there and never reach any hospital or institution where formal research is conducted" ... "the problem may be either trivial and transient, or the first evidence of a prolonged and perhaps terminal illness throughout which the patient will be directly or indirectly under the care of his family doctor" ... "thus the onus for much medical research is with the general practitioner". He continued his support for our research in Canada even after his retirement, providing great encouragement and practical help (Canadian Practitioners Invited, 1958).

The 1959 Research Committee – London

In the following year, 1959, the chairman of the CFPC research committee was <u>Dr. W.R. (Bill) Fraser</u>, of London,

Ontario.   Members of the committee were all from London, except for <u>Dr. R.M. (Reg) Anderson</u> of Oakville. He was possibly the only one with any research experience because of his job as medical director of the Mead Johnson Company. The others were <u>Dr. Gavin Hamilton</u>, <u>Dr. H.G. Fletcher</u>, <u>Dr. E.S. Jeffery</u>, and <u>Dr. F.F.R. Boyes</u>.   Mead Johnson had provided a grant of $5,000 per year, which was to be used for an educational program with no stipulation that it must be used for drug studies.   The College decided to allocate the money to a Research Fund for the development of a program of research in general practice.   A register of general practitioners interested in research had about fifty names.   Monthly meetings, held in the board room of St. Joseph's Hospital in London, Ontario, included some members of the Faculty of Medicine of the University of Western Ontario as advisors.

Topics appropriate for study included:

- specified areas in epilepsy
- febrile illness during pregnancy
- consequences of vaginal bleeding during the first two trimesters
- diabetes
- rheumatic fever after streptococcal infection
- the incidence of serious automobile accidents among patients with conditions alleged to increase the risks.

This list is an example to show that there was no lack of ideas for studies.   Indeed, it is likely that every family doctor in the country could come up with at least one valid question which has arisen during his time in practice.   Our problem was not a lack of ideas, but a lack of the requirements for turning the ideas into useful studies - especially the training in research methods, the time, the expense, and confidence in the importance of our contributions.

For some, the Mead Johnson grant might provide for development of a project to the stage where an application for money could be submitted to a major granting agency, thereby providing a great help over the first hurdle.

Deterrents

Major reasons for the relative lack of studies undertaken listed in the 1961 annual report, were:

- lack of experience in research
- lack of confidence that it was worthwhile
- lack of credibility, with no established record of successful studies or a substantial body of research in the field
- lack of support or appreciation, from partners or colleagues or from some university research consultants
- perceived lack of time, within a busy practice
- difficulty in obtaining funds

Encouragements

Major encouragements to overcome the obstacles included:

- a progressive increase in recognition and support by the College
- advice and personal contacts with members of the RCGP
- examples of studies by Canadians slowly coming to light
- occasional grants from the National Department of Health and Welfare for individual or group studies
- support from some university experts

Studies underway were:

- a national survey of phenylketonuria (Partington, M.W., 1964). Three cases were confirmed in 4,334 babies, and two were probable
- the use of antibiotics in prophylaxis in measles
- a tuberculin skin testing program

The 1963 Research Committee - Kingston

In 1963, the committee in London was dissolved and a new one was formed at Kingston, with Dr. M.C. Trotter as chairman and Dr. Reg Anderson continuing as secretary. The annual report in 1964 stated that "It had been abundantly demonstrated in the five years of the committee's existence in London that it was futile to hope for any results from a program designed to support clinical research by members of the College. As we pointed out in this report last year, general practitioners in Canada are not interested in clinical research".

It was noted that during the previous twelve months there was not a single enquiry about clinical topics. However, grants were provided to University of Alberta students, under Dr. Stanley Greenhill, for several studies initiated in 1963 and 1964:

- A comparison of city and rural practitioners. (Greenhill, S. & Singh, H.J., 1964 and 1965).
- Some Differences Between Patients Seen in Practitioners' Offices and those Admitted to Teaching Hospitals. (Greenhill , S. & Watts, P., 1964).
- A Critical Evaluation of a Family Study Program. (Greenhill, S. & Atkinson, M., 1964).
- How Important is a Hospital Bed to a General Practitioner? (Greenhill, S. & Kolotyluk , K., 1965).

Grants to other universities included support for:

- Attitudes of Medical Students to Family Practice. R.C.A. Hunter, M.D. and John Mount, B.Sc., McGill University (a three-year study).
- The Medical Student, the Family Physician Preceptor, and the Preceptor Program. J.H. Read, M.D. and Gary Lloyd at Queen's University.

Two other studies were mentioned - a quantitative survey of the therapeutic work done by physicians in St. Joseph's Hospital, Victoria, B.C., and a survey of the practices of rural, urban, and intermediately-located general practitioners in British Columbia by Dr. Peter Postuk in Duncan, B.C.

At the annual meeting of the College, the treasurer, Dr. Garth Diehl, was disturbed that the research committee had authority to spend the research grant as it saw fit, without the approval of the Board. He called for an annual audit of the books of the committee.

The following year, 1965, it was reported that seven studies had been completed by senior medical students and at least five would be published. More were planned for the summer of 1965; several other projects were suitable but could not be financed. Projects initiated included:

- The Role of the Public Health Nurse and other Social Services in Family Practice. D.A. Hutchison and R. Brennan, U.W.O.
- A Comparison of an Urban and a Rural Practice. J.J. Day, M.D. and R. Lewis, U. of Ottawa.
- A Descriptive Study of Injuries Involved in Sports, as seen by the General Practitioner. J. Read, M.D. and I. Arnold, Queens U.
- Comparison of Pattern and Range of Practice of a Three-man Group in a Large City (Vancouver) with that of a Similar Group in a Small Town (Castlegar). (Bartel, G.G., 1970).
- The Establishment of a Computer Program designed to provide ongoing data on the educational advancement of medical personnel in Alberta. Dr. S. Greenhill, Dr. S. Kling and G.J. McMurtry, U. of Alberta.
- A Study of the Variations in the Type of Work and the Workload of General Practitioners and the Relation of these Variations to their Place and Type of Practice. Dr. S. Greenhill and R. Zuege, U. of Alberta.
- The Influence of Social Characteristics of the Family on the Use of Medical Practitioners and Health Services. J.J. Day, M.D. and C. Beaudry, U. of Ottawa.
- Women in Family Practice. (Trenholme, M., 1967). As a medical student in Toronto, Trenholme conducted a mail survey of women doctors across Canada, as a summer

project. There were about 230 in general practice, with a wide range of interests and work loads.

The above list is presented in detail to show the degree of interest generated among medical students by their faculty, especially Dr. Stanley Greenhill at the U. of Alberta.

In 1966, several of the above projects were continuing, and several were added to the list:

- The Influence of Resident Mobility on the Utilization of Health Services. J.J. Day, U. of Ottawa.
- The statistical Significance of General Practitioner Loss over the Past Ten Years(Part a). To Obtain Accurate Personal Knowledge of the Reasons behind Decisions Made (Part b). L.M. Cathcart, M.D., B.C. Chapter, Research Committee.
- Tetanus Toxoid Recording System. Dr. D. Smith, London, Ontario.
- Psychiatry in Family Practice. Dr. J.A. Collyer, Leamington, Ontario (Collyer, J.A., 1968).

Some of the studies which were not supported, because of lack of grant money, showed other areas of relevance to family practice:

- A cooperative study of the natural history of disease in the offices of general practitioners. Dr. R.C. Harrison, U. of Alberta.
- A study of outpatient services and the participation of general practitioners. Dr. L.L. Morgan, Saint John, N.B.

"It was further reported by the committee that, in future, all research monies will be kept at the central office and made available to the research committee when required."   It was noted that Dr. D.G. Fish, Research Associate of the Association of Canadian Medical Colleges, had accepted an invitation to act as a consultant to the Committee on Research.

In his annual report to the College Board of Directors in 1967, Dr. Merrill Trotter mentioned again the major problem of limited financial resources. Funds were provided primarily by Mead Johnson of Canada Limited, augmented by moderate assistance from College finances. However, he was able to list four projects approved for grants of $1,200 each:

1. "A Study of the Major Health Problems in Children Attending a Family Practice Unit", by Dr. R.G. McAuley, McMaster University Hospital, Hamilton, Ontario.

2. "The Management of Obesity in Family Practice during Childhood and Adolescence", by Dr. John Read of Queen's University and Dr. K.G. Greller of Kingston, Ontario.

3. "Certain Aspects of Hospital Practice to Demonstrate the Part Played by the General Practitioner in the Care of his Patients", by Dr. J.A. Fowler and Dr. W.A. Falk, of Victoria, B.C. (Fowler, J.A., 1973).

4. "Why do Doctors Remain in General Practice?", by Dr. Conrad McKenzie, of Vancouver, B.C.

The last two projects were to be supported by College funds, apart from the research committee.

The report then announced that Dr. James A. Collyer, of London, had agreed to assume the chairmanship of the committee.

Some good examples

Several studies were reported in the Canadian Family Physician in 1968. Dr. James A. Collyer, then in Leamington, Ontario, wrote a detailed report on a study of 53 consecutive psychiatric patients (Collyer, J.A., 1968). Also in Leamington, Dr. James A. Taylor reported on the working hours of the general practitioner over a six-month period in 1967. This study, sponsored by the CFPC Research Committee, was considered "an outstanding example of how many of us might begin to study what we actually do in practice, as distinct from what we think we do". Taylor demonstrated several important essentials in starting any type of research - "Keep it simple, keep it short, and get it done. The most profound study in the world is of little use if it is not well-written and published" (Taylor, J.A., 1968).

A student research project in Ontario by Dr. Ian Arnold and Dr. Robert Steele, sponsored by the CFPC, described types of accidents and seasonal variations, as well as the role of the general practitioner in prevention and management. The period studied was from August, 1964, to May, 1965 (Arnold, I.M.F., 1968).

An exploratory study of twelve general practitioners, organized by Steele, Krause, and Smith, of Queens University, was supported by a Public Health Research Grant from the Department of National Health and Welfare (Steele, R., 1968).

The 1967 Research Committee - London

In 1967, the College started a major commitment to research when it appointed Dr. Jim Collyer as chairman of the research committee. Dr. Collyer was an energetic, innovative, and persuasive enthusiast, who had already been involved in projects in his own practice in Leamington, Ontario and then in London, Ontario. He could see the need for the College to make a coordinated effort to encourage and support potential researchers across the country. It should provide a source of advice and some practical help in finding needed resources.

At first he formed a nucleus committee in the London area, including Drs. A.T. Hunter, C.T. Lamont, K.E. Gay, P.B. Stein, and G. Pratt. The nucleus committee was expanded to create the National Research Advisory Committee by the addition of nineteen experts from departments of the University of Western Ontario, covering areas which were relevant:

- Preventive Medicine & Epidemiology: Dr. Carol Buck, Dr. Edgar J. Love, Dr. K. Stavarsky, Dr. J. Thurlow, and Dr. D. Hutchison

- Medicine: Dr. Donald Bondy, Dr. John Thompson, & Dr. Peter Rechnitzer.
- Obstetrics & Gynecology: Dr. J. Walters.
- Ophthalmology: Dr. R. T. Collyer.
- Pharmacology: Dr. C.W. Gowdy and Dr. John Parker.
- Anatomy: Dr. H.J. Hollenberg.
- Biochemistry: Dr. Milton Haines.
- Psychology: Dr. Bernie Portis, social psychologist, and Dr. Morris Schore, research consultant.
- Social Sciences: Mrs. Beryl Hall, divorce worker in Family and Children's Service.
- Computer Science: Mr. A.G. Wilford.
- Mathematics: Dr. T. Wonnacutt.

In his 1968 report, Dr. Collyer described well the opportunities for research in family practice, where every physician is a walking gold mine of experience which should be passed on to other physicians and the community. Because few have been trained in research methods, the National Committee aimed to encourage all members to record their experiences, and also to assist them with the technical means of designing, recording, and evaluating their work.

He emphasized that "On a broader scale, if this College is ever to justify its existence as an academic body, and its inclusion in the circles of those who decide on matters concerning medical education, it is time that we began to substantiate and justify our claims of clinical competence. We must begin to show that the Family Physician should not be continued merely because he is there, but because he has his own area of competence in which he does better than other physicians and for which he is uniquely suited."

Services planned by the committee included: a mailing advisory service, for helping to plan and initiate projects; statistical assistance; editorial assistance; and an index of family practice researchers with their special interests.

1969 – A National Research Committee Conference

The College supported Collyer in his plan to arrange a session in London, to which members from each province would be invited with the intention of encouraging more research activity in all chapters of the College. This organizational meeting took place January 17 and 18, 1969, at the University of Western Ontario, hosted by Professor Ian McWhinney's Subdepartment of Family Medicine and the Dean of Medicine, Dr. Douglas Bocking. Financial support came from a variety of sources (see Appendix 1 for program and list of delegates, supporters, and observers).

In his annual report to the Board, in April, 1969, Dr. Collyer described the enthusiasm of the organizers and delegates. On the first day, after introductory talks by Drs. McWhinney, Collyer, and Falk, there were small group discussions of four large topics - organization, financing, services, and projects. The next morning Dr. Collyer led a plenary session to consider recommendations to the board for a proposed constitution of the research committee with a national representation. In the afternoon, Dr. Paul Stein, of the nucleus committee, presented the results of the morning discussions and recommendations. The meeting closed with our special guest, Dr. Ian Watson, describing some of the work done by the RCGP and by himself. He had been actively involved with the research in general practice in Britain and had served as chairman of the research committee and later as president of the RCGP. He was invited to provide an overview and critique of the meeting. He ended with a challenge to the College to begin its task of critically studying our clinical work, our organization, and the natural history of illness as seen in family practice.

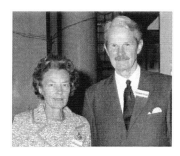

Dr. Ian and Carol Watson. Ian was the special guest at the Jan. 1969 meeting in London, Ontario

1969 – National Research Committee

After the board meeting in April, the committee was changed to include a member from each province. This was a truly national committee of general practitioners who had an active interest in research, although it lacked members from the Yukon or the Northwest Territories. It consisted of:

Dr. Jim Collyer, London, ON, Chairman
Dr. Laurie Zeilig, Toronto, ON, Secretary
Dr. John Ross, Placentia, NF
Dr. Iain MacPherson, Halifax, NS
Dr. Keith Ellis, Hunter River, PEI
Dr. Arthur Van Wart, Fredericton, NB
Dr. Alex Burton, Mount Royal, PQ
Dr. Alan MacFarlane, Hamilton, ON
Dr. Hugh Fairley, St. Vital, MN
Dr. Alan Clews, Saskatoon, SK.
Dr. Grant Mills, Calgary, AB
Dr. Bill Falk, Victoria, B.C.
Dr. John Z. Garson, Saskatoon, SK (co-opted)
Dr. Robert Westbury, Calgary, AB (co-opted)

The start of a national recording service

Shortly after the meeting in London, Dr. Collyer conducted a national survey, sending a postcard to all college members asking about their recent experience with influenza, as defined on the card. The response by about 1,500 members showed the potential value of information from the front lines. It can be processed more quickly than by the traditional public health reporting system. A willingness to participate in future studies was indicated by 90% of respondents, providing for each province a list of potential contributors to local, provincial, or national projects (Collyer, J.A., 1970). This demonstration of interest encouraged further steps to develop a national recording system. The College board approved the concept of an Illness Observation Unit (I.O.U.) which would collect reports from practices across the country, to study patterns of selected illnesses. One outcome of this idea was the Viral Watch, for which a recorder in each participating province submitted periodic reports to a provincial recorder, such as Dr. Michael Tarrant in Calgary, Alberta, and Dr. Peter Hoogewerf in Abbotsford, B.C. Data were processed by the College Research Unit.

The concept of reporting by a group of recorders was first tried in Saskatchewan, where Dr. John Garson conducted a five-week study of three illnesses of current interest (including mononucleosis and influenza-like illness). His wife, Ruth, contacted recorders weekly by phone, to ensure continuing cooperation, establishing a friendly link with recorders. Participants submitted a report card every week, or reported by phone. This study was financed by "money stolen from the household budget", a method advocated by Dr. Pinsent.

Workshops

The committee embarked on a program to stimulate interest among general practitioners across Canada, and to provide opportunities for them to learn some of the basic requirements of doing research (see Chapter 4). Substantial support from the College provided a series of workshops on methods of research after the initial session in London in 1969. In September of 1970, the 'Muskoka Workshop', at the Sherwood Inn on Muskoka Lake in Ontario, provided a great stimulus to those attending, many of whom have appeared in subsequent studies and reports. Guest faculty consisted of major contributors to the research work of the Royal College of General Practitioners. This workshop was the first of three national sessions, with delegates invited from all provinces. Two more national workshops were held, in Banff, Alberta and Chester, Nova Scotia (details in Appendix 2).

One of the first provincial workshops was held in Halifax, Nova Scotia, on October 18, 1969, organized by the provincial research committee chairman, Dr. Iain MacPherson. After the January 1969 meeting in London, a nucleus committee was formed with Dr. MacPherson, Dr. Eugene Nurse, and Dr. James Fraser. They stimulated the formation of six regional committees in Nova Scotia with corresponding members who were chosen because of ability, interest, and willingness to become involved. There was also an advisory committee which included several resource persons who were not general practitioners. Several papers at the workshop described the basics of research, including the problems. Dr. Donald Brown described his experience with studies of papanicolau smears over an eight-year period. He averaged one carcinoma-in-situ for every 97 smears, in patients with an average age of 36, and there were three invasive carcinomas in patients averaging 43 years of age.

Provincial workshops were held in other places, including Harrison Hot Springs, BC, Banff, Winnipeg, Halifax and Moncton, NB in 1972; Harrison Hot Springs and Winnipeg in 1973; Victoria, BC in 1974. Workshops were also held in Duncan, BC; Regina, Saskatchewan; Toronto. Many of these had the benefit of visiting resource persons such as Dr. Donald Crombie, Dr. Bent Bentsen, Dr. Keith Hodgkin and Dr. Ian McWhinney, all of whom had extensive experience in family medicine research.

The National Research Committee report of March 1970 described the progress following the January 1969 meeting in London. Provincial research committees had been organized in three provinces, adding to those already in place in Newfoundland and B.C., while others were in the process of forming. A regular Research Newspage had been appearing in the Canadian Family Physician. A proposal for a major project in clinical research was presented by Dr. Iain MacPherson, to establish an antenatal score system in Nova Scotia, to assess the risk factors and to improve the results of obstetrical care. This project was to be discussed at the workshop on research methods at Muskoka in September.

As in most committees, there was some turnover of memberships. Resigning members were replaced by:

- In April, 1969, Dr. Don Rae of Portage la Prairie, MN and Stuart McDonald of Charlottetown, PEI
- In January 1970, new members were; Murray Nixon of St. John, NB; Henry Dirks of Winnipeg, MN; and Larry McNally from Quebec.
- In September 1970 Mel Parsons of Glovertown, NF, joined. Jim Collyer resigned as chairman, to be replaced by Bill Falk of Victoria, B.C..
- John Sumner of Maple Ridge, BC, and Stan Sinclair from Quebec were added in March 1971. Claude Labelle from Calgary, AB, and David Road from Regina, SK, joined in September 1971.
- In 1972, Paul Minc from Ontario and Michael Tarrant from Calgary, AB, joined.
- In October 1973 Drs. Fred DeManuele of Toronto, ON, Brian Dixon-Warren from Maple Ridge, BC and Douglas Robb from New Brunswick replaced previous members.
- In 1974, John O'Connor of Ontario was added to the committee. Bill Falk resigned as chairman, to be replaced by Alan Clews of Victoria.

The diverse personalities, length of experience, and areas of practice helped to maintain the level of enthusiasm and activity in the committee over its developing years. It will be noted that most of the committee members were in private practice at that time.

Dr. Robert Westbury

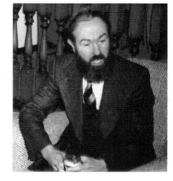

Bob, in his usual perceptive style, has recently described the feeling of friendship and cooperation in the committee.

"Those of us on the committee saw ourselves as a small band of missionaries in a hostile land, and so we were drawn very close to each other, to the extent that other members of the C.F.P.C. tended to think of us as a sort of club. In retrospect, this may have been a fair allegation, but our intense bonding gave us the energy to do some useful things for the nascent science of Family Practice at that time. We did all the usual things that committees need to do, but at the same time our enthusiasm was raised to fever pitch at each meeting for the many tasks that we had to do between meetings, and our efforts were spurred on by a desire not to let down our friends."

Much of the research activity has been reported in the Canadian Family Physician (CFP), which has been supportive of the research efforts, especially in the early years with editors David Wood and Margaret McCaffery. In spite of this support, when the CFP published its Twenty-fifth Anniversary Issue in 1979, there was practically no mention of research in the articles about the early years of the College, as pointed out by Livingston in his critique of that issue. However, the May 1973 issue had been devoted to research articles by Canadians. Unfortunately, the CFP was not included in the Index Medicus, so that its relevant papers might be listed only in publications specifically aimed at recording studies in family medicine, such as the comprehensive list prepared by the Royal College of General Practitioners. A Canadian list was needed, and was soon produced, as described in Chapter 6.

Summation

Although the College had an expressed interest in research from its beginning, and tried to stimulate its members into doing research, acceptance in the field was slow. It seemed that the top-down approach was not working, and that it needed workers at the "coal-face" to develop the needed curiosity about what they were doing. Most of the early projects started by individuals were small, but covered topics useful in practice and presumably of satisfaction to the researchers. The extent and speed of interest increased when Dr. Jim Collyer became chairman of the National Research Committee and worked hard to establish it on a national basis. As always, the cost of operating a national committee was in the foreground, but the College accepted Collyer's ideas and supported his plan for selling college members on the fact that they were capable of doing research, and that it was a necessary activity to provide a sound basis for family medicine. The resulting succession of national and provincial workshops supported by the College attracted many members who have since contributed greatly to research and to publication of their findings.

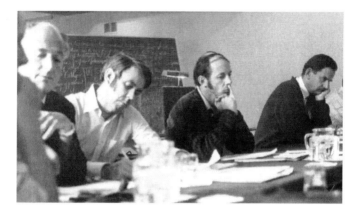

The 1971 research committee met at Banff, including
Drs. John Garson, Jim Collyer, Alan Clews, Bill Falk
Photo by Ruth Garson

Chapter 4

Training for Research

In the early years, much of the research done by individual general practitioners was by methods improvised or learned by reading. The first organized national efforts in Canada to provide systematic training in the principles of research were at the workshops sponsored by the College of Family Physicians of Canada. At both national and provincial levels, those attending were presented with the basic needs in planning projects, such as methodology and hypothesis formulation. They were also shown how to proceed with their ideas, step by step. Discussion often continued after the scheduled sessions had finished, in the dining room and sometimes the swimming pool. The attendance was usually about thirty to forty students, at different levels of interest and experience. Some contributed to the teaching. Visiting experts from Britain, who were our role models, learned about the different problems in Canada, especially the effects of long distances between centres with the costs and time of travel and the need for good communication between meetings.

The College's Workshops

Following the organizational meeting in London in January, 1969, the expanded research committee started on plans to provide more opportunities for general/family practitioners to learn research methods.

Muskoka Workshop

At the first national workshop, at the Sherwood Inn in the Muskoka Lake district north of Toronto, four prominent general practitioners came from Britain to serve as consultants and contributors for the three days of the sessions. They had all been involved in research in the Royal College of General Practitioners since its early days, and collectively had extensive experience in personal and group research.

- Dr. Robin Pinsent, Research Advisor to the Birmingham General Practice Research Unit, had his practice surgery in his home and conducted some of his research there.
- Dr. Donald Crombie, who worked closely with Dr. Pinsent, was Director of the General Practice Research Unit in Birmingham.
- Dr. Clifford Kay, who practised half-time in Manchester, spent the other half of his time conducting the large national study of oral contraceptives – the first study to show that the risk of harmful effects was extremely low.
- Dr. Ekke Kuenssberg was in a group practice in Edinburgh, where he developed a family register of diseases. He showed the tendency of members of a family to have similar illness patterns, not necessarily just infections.

Each of these visitors had also been active in the early days of the local and national bodies of the Royal College of General Practitioners, in a variety of positions.

The enthusiasm generated by the Muskoka Workshop gave the research movement in Canada a tremendous boost. After the meeting, Drs. Pinsent and Kay travelled west, contributing to provincial research committees in Winnipeg, Regina, Calgary, Vernon, Vancouver, and Victoria. Similarly Drs. Crombie and Kuenssberg travelled east to consult with local and provincial committees.

The Muskoka workshop was special with recognition of the importance of family support for researchers. Much of their work was done on a small budget and in spare time, with help of family members. Some participants were accompanied by spouses (at their own expense) to sit in on some of the sessions and to enjoy the beauty of the lakes with autumn colours. Contacts made gave them a better understanding of the aspirations and needs of the research committee, as well as some of their achievements (see Appendix 2).

Banff Workshop

With the precedents of the London Assembly and the Muskoka Workshop, another national workshop was held in Banff, Alberta, in September 1971. It was organized by Drs. Robert Westbury and Michael Tarrant, of Calgary. Both had been recording diagnoses and patient encounters in their group practice. They set up a poster display, showing research methods, as well as the results of their studies and those of other family physicians. As at Muskoka, speakers at the workshop sessions covered the basic principles of research, with examples from practice (see Appendix 2).

Before the workshop there was a meeting of the National Research Committee, which usually tried to make maximum use of the time together, to economize on travel costs.

Chester Workshop

Because of the expense and time involved in travel, most of those attending the Banff workshop were from the west. Therefore a third national workshop was held to accommodate members in the east. The provincial committee organizing this session had learned from the experience of holding the provincial workshop in Halifax, in October, 1969. It was chaired by Dr. Iain MacPherson of Halifax, chairman of the provincial research committtee (MacPherson, I.G., 1970). He also organized the national workshop in May 1972, at Chester, Nova Scotia, featuring presentations on basic principles of research by members of the national and provincial committees (see Appendix 2).

Interest from the U.S.A.

During the Chester workshop there was a surprise visit by two guests from Richmond, Virginia. They had just come from the inaugural meeting of the North American Primary Care Research Group (NAPCRG), the first organized approach to family practice research in the U.S.A. Dr. Maurice Wood had moved from Britain to be the first Professor of Family Medicine at the Medical College of Virginia in Richmond. Dr. Jack Froom was a U.S.A.

graduate who had practised as an internist before joining the Family Practice Department of the State University of New York in Rochester. They showed a tremendous enthusiasm for research, inflamed by their meeting in Virginia, and had a great interest in the work already accomplished by the Canadian College. NAPCRG developed quickly, in relation to the rate of growth of our organization in Canada. It soon became a dominant force in family medicine research in North America, and has included many Canadian members.

The national workshops were expensive projects. The College supported travel and accommodation for those attending, so that the number of registrants was limited to about forty. The expectation was that those chosen to attend would maintain a continuing interest, by doing their own studies or by contributing to group projects. In the provincial chapters, workshops frequently became part of annual scientific assemblies. Eventually, more papers by family physicians were included in the scientific programs of provincial and national meetings of the College.

Health Care Evaluation Seminars

In 1970, there was a shortage of health care evaluators in Canada, and "large numbers of health care providers, administrators, and planners were attempting to evaluate specific programs without the benefit of training in or access to health care evaluation methods. It was against this background that the Health Care Evaluation Seminar Program was conceived" (Baskin, M. et al, 1980). This program used a large resource manual with a comprehensive list of papers covering the many aspects of evaluation (Sackett, D.L., 1971). The manual, compiled at McMaster University by Dr. David Sackett as project director, served as a focus for each of the thirteen seminars, evolving to a third edition in 1978.

The five-day seminars, at thirteen centres across Canada, provided tutors to work closely with participants, with a ratio of two students to one tutor. There were about twelve tutors, and a range of 18 to 29 students. Students were selected from applicants who had projects in an early stage of development, with the objective of working with appropriate consultants throughout the week, to complete or advance the planning. Consultants were available from local universities and government offices, by appointment.

The cost of travel and accommodation for students and faculty were covered by the program.

Ottawa, Ontario, February 1973

My first contact with the program was attendance at the fourth seminar, held in Ottawa. Organized by Dr. John Last, it was aimed especially at family physicians. The twenty students were from a variety of disciplines: nursing, social work, administration, medicine – including thirteen family physicians. Details are in Appendix 3.

Victoria, B.C., November 1975

Appreciating the value of this type of intensive short program, the National Research Committee of the College wished to sponsor a seminar aimed primarily at family physicians who had already shown an interest and ability in research. With the help and advice of Pamela Poole, from the National Department of Health and Welfare, an application for support of a seminar was approved. Co-hosts and planners were Dr. Alan Clews, in private practice in Victoria and chairman of the National Research Committee, and Dr. Fred Demanuele from the family medicine teaching program at the Sunnybrook Hospital in Toronto.

This seminar was a highly-significant milestone in the progress of the College in several ways: 1) Although various projects had been financed by the Department of Health and Welfare through the years, this was a major commitment to the College in support of its research aspirations. The plans and choice of participants were developed by the College research committee in consultation with the organizers of the series. 2) The tutors included several family physicians. 3) most of the participants were family physicians.

Each 'student' was assigned to a tutor. Each tutor had two students to work closely with during the week, for discussion of their projects and for suggestions of consultants who would be appropriate for their projects. As well, there were opportunities for appointments with consultants from the list.

Of the twenty-four students in Victoria, seventeen were general practitioners/family doctors. The other seven were from the disciplines of Social Work, Nursing, and Psychology. The family doctors were at various levels of practice, from one in a residency, some in private practice or clinics, and others in university teaching programs. Their experience in research ranged from very little to extensive.

Gradual progress

On a smaller but more frequent scale was the increasing inclusion of research sessions and papers at provincial and national meetings of the College, and the provincial workshops as described in Chapter 3.

There was more frequent publication of research results or advice in the Canadian Family Physician and the Canadian Medical Association Journal. A broader perspective was provided by meetings and publications of WONCA and NAPCRG.

The series of workshops and seminars through the early seventies was intended to provide family physicians with some skills and confidence in their ability to contribute useful research. The success of these efforts is difficult to measure, but the following years have shown a tremendous increase in the number of projects conducted and results published by family physicians. This increase might be coincidental, but the names of some of those attending the training sessions have appeared prominently in publications since then.

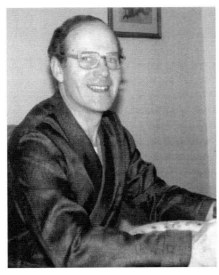

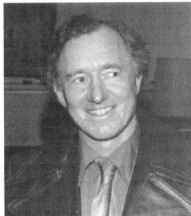

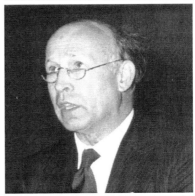

Top left - Dr. Clifford Kay,
   in Calgary
Top right - Dr. Donald Crombie,
   1973, after Harrison Workshop
Right- Dr. Ekke Kuenssberg

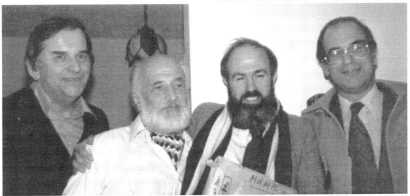

1982 in Calgary : (left to right)
Drs. Bill Falk, John Garson, Robert Westbury, and Mike Tarrant

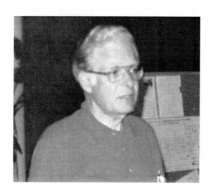

Dr. Kerr White

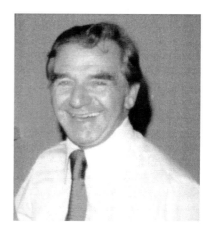

Dr. Maurice Wood

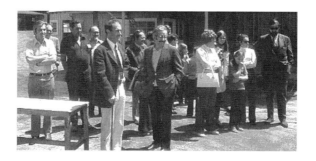

During a break at Chester - group includes
Drs. Bob Westbury and Jack Froom in front,
and Dr. Doug Robb at the far right

Chapter 5

The University

When I was planning to go into general practice, while in a rotating internship at the Vancouver General Hospital in 1950, it seemed that some extra training would be a good idea. The only opportunities available for non-specialists were called general practice residencies. There were four in North America, all in the U.S.A. I chose the closest one, the small Columbus Hospital in Seattle (now called the Saint Frances Xavier Cabrini), where I was one of two residents for six months, and then the only resident for the last six months. We also had six live-in medical students to examine new patients, write histories and take first call. There was one intern to share second call. The hospital work was the main source of exposure to general practitioners. I was involved in all services for the full year, usually at least half the day in surgery. There was no time planned in general practice offices or home visits. My only contact with research was a required project, reviewing records of wound dehiscence and scanning the literature. I vaguely remember that Vitamin C seemed to be beneficial.

Teaching of Family Medicine

One of the problems faced by the College of General Practice of Canada was the need to define an area of expertise which could be taught. After much deliberation, at the 1967 Annual Scientific Assembly in Vancouver the name was changed to "The College of Family Physicians of Canada". This move led to the adoption of 'Family Medicine' as the academic basis for family practice and the focus for future research to show what was involved in family practice.

Chapter 5

The first departments of family medicine

The College wished to start a teaching program for residents in family practice. In 1966 it supported London, Ontario, and Calgary, Alberta, as the experimental sites.

At the University of Western Ontario (generally known as Western), Dr. Ian McWhinney became their Professor of Family Medicine in 1968. He had already established a reputation for research in a group practice in England. His department at Western was involved in research from the beginning, and has continued to be a major contributor to research and teaching in Canada.

In Calgary, before there was a medical school, the family medicine residency was started at the same time as London, at the Calgary General Hospital. Dr. Tom Saunders came into the program, followed by many of his patients. He was its head until the medical school was formed and Dr. Morris Gibson became the first professor of family medicine. The research work of the department received a boost when Dr. George McQuitty joined, using his practice in Cochrane as a teaching practice attached to the university. While carrying a heavy workload of patient care and teaching, and later as head of the department, he worked on a major computer program to record diagnoses, tests, treatments and outcomes. It was just starting to produce results at the time of his sudden death in 1979 while cross-country skiing. Nobody in the department was capable of continuing his work. He had written that the knowledge and understandiing of the patient, built up over time, was the unique field of family practice that should be emphasized. (McQuitty, G.D.H., 1973).

All medical schools followed the first two

Eventually, all medical schools in Canada had departments of family medicine. At first, the focus of the new departments had to be on teaching and patient care. Local practitioners came into the units with their patients and worked with the residents to provide the usual care. Some general practitioners who had acquired research experience in private practice were attracted into the teaching departments. Prominent among these were Dr. Jim Collyer and Dr. Paul Newell at Western; Dr. Michael Tarrant and Dr. Wayne Elford at Calgary; Dr. Ron McAuley at McMaster and Dr. John Ross at Memorial University in Newfoundland.

Family physicians recruited to the universities bridged a gap between practising family doctors and university professors, because of their previous work in the community and their contacts among their colleagues. They helped to obtain cooperation in studies which needed a large patient population and multiple recorders. They also served as consultants or partners in projects originated in the community or by the provincial College chapters.

Research

The need for acceptance

A major obstacle to the acceptance (by specialists in the university) of Family Medicine as a discipline was the lack of a clearly-defined body of knowledge and a large enough research background to substantiate it. (Some critics wondered how well the body of knowledge for each other specialty had been defined). While departments of family medicine were trying to become established, their first priority was the practical teaching of family medicine residents. Research was generally secondary, acknowledged as a need but given low priority when resources were allocated. Encouragement was given by some departments of community medicine, which seemed to have a better appreciation of the potential of family medicine research than did the departments of family medicine.

One of the earliest efforts to develop a research function in the B.C. Chapter of the College had been the formation of a research committee in 1964. Dr. George Gibson, of Chilliwack, when appointed as chairman, started by planning a study on hypertension. When he approached a noted hypertension expert for advice, he was told firmly that general practitioners should not be doing research. At the time, there were no other visible sources of help, so his idea quietly succumbed.

Encouragement

Fortunately, there were more encouraging responses from others who were willing to give advice or practical help. At U.B.C., Dr. Cortland Mackenzie, a former general practitioner who was then head of the Department of Health Care and Epidemiology, worked with Dr. Peter Postuk to analyze some of the data from eight years of recording in his group practice in Duncan. This collaboration resulted in publication of a report on two years of data (Postuk, P. D., 1969). Also at U.B.C., Dr. Don Williams, who conducted the program of continuing education, was an enthusiastic supporter of education and research in general practice, and encouraged early activity by the B.C. Chapter of the College.

In other universities, many of the faculty were supportive of general practice research and available as members of local and national research committees. Dr. Ed Love, at Western and later at the University of Calgary, was involved as a tutor at National Health Grant Seminars. He also tried to encourage work by family physicians in his capacity as head of the Department of Community Health Sciences in Calgary. Dr. Stanley Greenhill, at the U. of Alberta, worked with medical students for several years when the Mead Johnson funds which were available had not been requested by physicians in practice and were allocated to Dr. Greenhill's students. At McMaster Univerity, Dr. David Sackett and a group of family doctors in the faculty stimulated production of many studies.

Dr. Harding leRiche, at the University of Toronto, advocated the study of common diseases, their management and outcomes. He questioned the use of ancillary workers to take histories, feeling that doctors would be better at analyzing and studying the patient's unstated complaints and anxieties (leRiche, W.H., 1975). He counted entries in the world-wide list maintained by the RCGP librarian, Margaret Hammond, (Hammond, M., 1971), and identified the small number of Canadian research projects included in that list.

In the U.S.A. one of the earliest advocates for research and education in family medicine was an epidemiologist, Dr. Kerr White (White, K.L., 1961). His major article on 'The Ecology of Medical Care' included a diagram showing the small number of patients from the total population who were available for much of the research done by specialists in teaching hospitals – where most of the teaching of medical students was done. He called for more research to be done by general practitioners, who saw the patients who were not admitted to teaching hospitals. In speaking to the 59th Annual Congress on Medical Education in 1963, he outlined the reasons for involving some general practitioners in teaching units, and the need to have time allotted for research and reflection (White, K.L., 1963). Since then, all Canadian medical schools have established departments of family medicine, and most have encouraged or required an emphasis on research. However, the time provided for reflection was harder to define and protect in the face of the need for patient care and student and resident teaching.

One major source of support was found at Western, where Dr. Jim Collyer enlisted a large number of consultants for the National Research Committee, covering all relevant disciplines. In the ground-breaking meeting at Western in January, 1969, support was given by deans of medicine: at Western, Dr. Douglas Bocking; at Ottawa, Dr. Lussier; at Calgary, Dr. W. Cochrane; at McMaster, Dr. John Evans; at U.B..C. Dr. John McCreary (See Appendix 1). It is likely that encouragement and support were given by individuals in other universities for other meetings and research efforts.

Survey of patient and doctor attitudes

In 1970, the B.C. Chapter of the College formed a Lay Advisory Committee, to obtain opinions about the health care available in Vancouver. Terms of reference were 1) to consider the medical needs of the consumer and 2) availability of medical services as they relate to the College's position concerning education and manpower.

A study was organized and run in 1971 by the B.C. Chapter and Morton Warner, a sociologist in the Department of Health Care and Epidemiology at U.B.C. Lay contributors were a combination of young and old, with a variety of experiences and skills. They were interested in several areas – the organization of practice, the contact with the doctor, and the role of the family physician in arranging for help by other disciplines.

Among the results, some showed a large difference between the views of patients and of G.P.'s. Patients showed acceptance of a trained nurse to do some procedures, such as blood pressure measurement, ear syringing, nutritional teaching, and medical histories. Physicians would delegate more functions, except in the taking of histories and pap smears. For treating all members of a family, 75% of physicians thought it was important, compared with 62% of patients. Routine checkups were favoured more by patients than by physicians, although only 4% of each group thought they should never be done.

One finding of importance was the making of house calls by 99% of family physicians, a fact that might suprise politicians and economists who maintained that house calls were not done any more.

During the previous twelve months, 11.8% of patients had had no contact with the family doctor.

A surprising response was 85% of family physicians indicating that research was important to personal satisfaction with practice. Also, 93% would leave practice if offered a full-time post in a medical school with the same or less income, and another 5% would leave for a greater income.

Non-medical liaison and help

Apart from the medical faculty, Dr. Harry Warren, Professor of Geology at U.B.C., wished to work with general practitioners. He had done extensive work in identifying differences of trace element distribution in soils and plants in various locations. From his findings, he had good reason to postulate that these differences might have some relationship to some diseases. He had many examples of suspicious coincidence, such as swayback in horses in pastures contaminated by pollution from smelters in Trail, B.C., as well as an apparent excess of cases of multiple sclerosis in Trail. He was careful not to go beyond the bounds of his expertise, and tried to create an effective working relationship with the B.C. Chapter of the College to plan an interdisciplinary study.

A grant application was prepared in 1973, with major support and input by Dr. Charles Laszlo, Ph.D., a National Health Scientist and Associate Director of the Division of Health Systems at U.B.C. He took on the onerous job of preparing the application on his computer. The proposed study was to show a difference in the incidence of multiple sclerosis in relation to the distribution of some trace elements in the environment, in two similar but geographically-separated towns. Sadly, the application was rejected by Health and Welfare Canada (twice), the Vancouver Foundation, and the B.C. Medical Services Foundation. The momentum for continuing was lost.

Summation

The above examples are not to be considered the only indications of support by university experts in various fields. It is quite likely that each university had individuals who had either helped or would have helped if asked. Many agreed to serve on the Advisory Committee formed by Jim Collyer in London. Many also contributed to the Health Care Evaluation Seminars. Some of our failures might have been a result of our inexperience at the time, or perhaps our lack of credibility because of a very short track record in conducting relatively large studies. However, we had to remember that with each effort we learned something useful which could be applied in future proposals.

It was said by some of The College hierarchy that the research committee was too Anglophile. In fact, the most inspiration and help came from the British contacts, especially after Dr. Robin Pinsent's visit to Montreal in 1964. There were no well-known research authorities in the newly-formed departments of family medicine in the medical schools, except for Dr. Ian McWhinney at Western, who had come from Stratford-upon-Avon in England. It seemed that many of the Canadian general practitioners who became active in research in the early days had trained in Britain, and it was certain that much of our best work came from that group. It was fair comment that the research activity was Anglocentric, also that much (or most) of it was done in private practices, before the medical schools became involved.

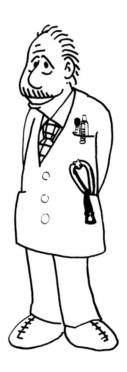

"I sometimes wonder if
what I am doing is right"

Chapter 6

Communications

When a question is posed, a hypothesis stated or a project started, it is with the assumption that there is an answer somewhere. Research is a process of communication, to find the answer and to report it in a form which can be understood and put to work to benefit our patients or the community at large. Often the findings of the day are proven to be wrong when further research produces different and better answers.

Communication, then as now, was vital to the conduct of research. Using and contributing to the literature was recognized as a basic need. Personal interaction, whether by meetings or through the mail, was necessary to coordinate and critique activities. In a large country, such as Canada, face-to-face meetings were expensive and could be held only on a limited basis.

Libraries

When the National Research Committee was formed, the Canadian literature of family medicine research was meager. The number of studies done was small, and those published in the Canadian Family Physician would not show up in a search of the Index Medicus (IM), which was generally accepted as the major reference for medical publications world-wide. Until the advent of computer access to the literature, a search meant long hours reading pages of fine print. In his survey of the literature in 1971 Michael Livingston found few original studies by general practitioners in Canada. He described nine case reports and twelve research articles published from 1957 to 1971, presumably listed in IM although two articles from the Canadian Family Physician were included in his list (Livingston, M.C.P., 1972). Livingston expanded on his list of researchers in a report in the Canadian Family Physician

(Livingston, M.C.P., 1974), a useful attempt to "rescue from obscurity the work of 21 Canadian family physician researchers in the period 1950-1970".

The Canadian Library of Family Medicine

One of the first activities of the new national research committee was the establishment of the Canadian Library of Family Medicine. It was the idea of Dr. Robert Westbury of Calgary, who worked on its organization and chaired the library committee. The library was given space in the medical library at Western, and was supported financially by the College. Rather than being a collection of books, it was set up as a reference centre to which College members from across Canada could write or phone to ask for reprints or literature searches on any topic. The references available included more than the Index Medicus, as the library aimed to include any publications relevant to family medicine. It was one of the early steps towards development of a much-needed academic base for family medicine. The first librarian was Mr. Ashford Johnson in 1972, succeeded by Dorothy Fitzgerald, and by Lynn Dunikowski. Other sources of information were described by Westbury (Westbury, R.C., 1970).

Medical schools

Just as the school at Western had a library which could accommodate the small library of family medicine, each medical school served the medical community as well as the students. As an example, even the library at U.B.C., one of the youngest medical schools, had an extensive collection of books and journals, as well as an archival section.

Medical organizations

As an example of a provincial service, the library of the B. C. College of Physicians and Surgeons has been available for many years, having evolved from the early establishment by the Vancouver Medical Association. This library was linked to local medical libraries throughout the province. The Victoria Medical Society library, another old one, has been helpful in providing references for this book. It has a collection of current and old journals, some of which are from the nineteenth century. It is likely that the other provinces have similar services available.

The library of the RCGP, mentioned above for its bibliography, is also a prime source of books and journals related to general practice. It has encouraged contact with family doctors from other countries, offering help to search the literature.

Personal

The large volume of material arriving because of membership in various organizations creates a problem of storage. A selection process was necesssary to preserve those which were considered most likely to be of interest in future, or to file tear-outs so they could be retrieved easily. Books also could be useful, although some clinical texts could be out-dated too soon while others have basic knowledge which remains pertinent. Some books had historical interest and value, according to the interests of the individual, and some had basic principles which stood the test of time.

Bibliographies

Various lists of research work done by general practitioners have been prepared. The following include the best available, and contain many more references than can be included with the examples chosen for this book. They show the range and breadth of subjects and of researchers.

The RCGP list

The best source of information about general practice projects was the library of the Royal College of General Practitioners, in London, England. The librarian, Margaret Hammond, maintained and published a record of general practice studies throughout the world. For years, this was the only reasonably complete list available for family medicine.

The ACGP Digest

The Australian College of General Practitioners published the Research Digest (Rowe, I.L., [Ed., 1968, 1972]), a list of studies done in Australia during the ten-year period up to 1968. An abstract was written for each entry. This was followed in 1972 by another list of recent projects. Some of these are descibed in Chapter 3, as examples, but the total number is overwhelming when we consider the size of the country and the relatively small population compared with other world powers.

Zaborenko

In 1968 Zaborenko and Zwell published a list of studies in general practice, most of which were from the U.S.A. or Britain (Zaborenko, L., 1968). Many were from the JRCGP, and most had been published since 1960. They noted that the number of publications in the 18-month period in which they were collecting data equalled the number in the preceding six years, and that many were from individual general practitioners reporting on their own practices. In a follow-up bibliography on training for family practice, they included many additonal references (Zwell, M.E., 1970).

Tenney

Another useful list of studies of the content of medical practice was compiled by Dr. James Tenney and published by Johns Hopkins University (Tenney, J.B., 1969).

RAP

The Research Awareness Publication (RAP) was another brainchild of Dr. Robert Westbury, who originated and produced an occasional current list of projects by Canadian family physicians. It appeared first in December, 1970. Seven issues were published at irregular intevals until August, 1976. Projects were listed according to category of research, in four main groups: epidemiological, organizational, clinical and therapeutic. RAP was unique in classifying projects also according to the stage of development: idea – planned – underway – completed - published – or abandoned. Successive issues showed progress from the idea stage to the final outcome (Westbury, R.C., 1971 and 1973). RAP included many more studies than I have listed as examples. Apart from those published, RAP showed many ideas which never proceeded to completion, although it showed topics which were considered to be important enough to be worth studying.

By 1976, the College had developed a research office at its headquarters in Toronto, and the listing of projects was taken over by research associate Daniel Brackstone, Ph.D. The general idea of RAP was continued and in 1980 was expanded into a new publication called *Family Medicine Research: a Current Canadian Index.*

FAMLI

Also in 1980, WONCA published the first edition of the *Family Medicine Literature Index* '(FAMLI), using the same format as Index Medicus, to provide a record of work done in any country. It would have been useful in the early years.

Journals

From its early days as a newsletter *Between Ourselves,* the RCGP record of the results of research by general practitioners was ahead, in time and scope, of any general practice journal in the world. The newsletter grew to become *The Journal of the Royal College of General Practitioners* (JRCGP), providing a medium for publishing papers from around the world. It is now called the *British Journal of General Practice.*

In Canada and the U.S.A., the general practice journals were publishing many articles by specialists, often in the how-to-do-it category, but little original research by family doctors. It seemed that the reason for a lack of published articles was the lack of research by general practitioners, along with failure to take the final step of preparing results suitably for publication. The *Canadian Family Physician* (CFP) was not listed in the Index Medicus, so there was a disincentive to submit research papers to it. However, after the research committee started its new approach in 1968, space was provided by the supportive editor, David Woods, for a monthly newspage to promote an interest in research. A latent interest became apparent when readership surveys gave the research newspage a consistently high rating. In time, more research papers were submitted by family physicians. Eventually the journal was listed in Index Medicus, possibly because of the increased number of research papers.

Other publications appeared, directed primarily at promoting and printing research reports by family practitioners. The *Journal of Family Practice* (JFP) in the U.S.A., was started by NAPCRG in 1978 and published monthly. As well as publishing studies in general practice, it produced useful special editions devoted to the general principles and methods of research, and to some of the basic studies of the content of family practice.

Examples of the work in other countries were published in journals such as the *American Family Physician* (AmFP) and the *Australian Family Physician* (AuFP), known originally as the *Annals of General Practice*.

The international *WONCA News,* which started in 1974, eventually was included in a new publication by Oxford University press, *Family Practice.* Along with general information about activities in family practice, WONCA News included reports on research by the many member countries.

Committee Activities

Even with all the literature available, there was still a need for face-to-face contacts at reasonable intervals, to allow for discussion and planning of objectives and projects. Nowadays the prevalence of aids such as fax machines, conference calls, and E-mail might reduce the need for meetings, but those things were not readily available in the early days.

Meetings

When Dr. Jim Collyer's new national committee took shape, with members from each province, the major benefit was the establishment of personal links between members. These were strengthened at two-day meetings of the committee, usually in Toronto. Each provincial member would report on developments, leading to a detailed discussion of progress. Plans to promote and assist research activity nationally as well as provincially were presented for critique and possible action. It was still necessary for the committee to convince the Board of the College, which had provided good support and encouragement, of its capabilities in research. Other committees of the College tended to undertake surveys and projects without using the potential benefit of advice from the research committee members, who might have benefited from the experience of evaluating plans.

An omnipresent problem in all Canadian committees was the size of the country. A British visitor to the Muskoka Workshop, Ruth Pinsent, wearily commented on a boat cruise "but there's so much of everything!". Communication in any form was expensive. The cost of airfare and accommodation for a two-day meeting of fifteen members required a large budget, and two meetings per year were the limit. It was necessary to conduct much of the work of the committee by mail, or by telephone. We could envy the relative ease of communication in Britain, where the small size of the country made meeting much easier. On the other hand, Australia had the same difficulty as Canada, with an even smaller population spread mostly over the southern portion of a large country, with its largest population centres in the east. In spite of the similar geographical problems, the Australian College had produced a large and useful body of research.

Some of the papers presented at workshops and scientific sessions of the College, NAPCRG and WONCA were published in 'proceedings' which were distributed to registrants but not usually published elsewhere. Many of these were based on recent research or works in progress, and were printed as abstracts rather than complete descriptions of the work. Discussions with the audience had the potential to improve a final publication or to improve the planning for a project.

Delphi

To help provide timely advice to those planning projects, a major initiative was undertaken by Dr. John Garson, of Saskatoon. He developed a postal network for long-range discussion of research proposals by family physicians, to provide a variety of informed feedback. This network, named Delphi, involved making and mailing copies of proposals to members of the national research committtee, with a request to study them and return a critique within a specified time.

To follow the theme of the Delphic Oracle, Dr. Garson was given the name 'Oribasius' in his communications with his widely-scattered team of minor oracles. The first project, started in December, 1970, was to give opinions and suggestions about the proposed Illness Observation Unit. The mnemonic 'IOU' was intended to indicate that we owe it to our patients to study their problems so that we might improve their treatment. This project went through a long process of planning, and eventually surfaced as the National Research System (NaReS). Over the next four years, opinions were requested by Delphi on a variety of projects, such as :

- Use of a Physician's Associate
- Package Programs, in cooperation with the Research Unit of the RCGP
- The Canadian Library of Family Medicine
- Family Life Education
- The Diagnostic Process
- Trace elements related to Morbidity
- Vitamin E in Coronary Heart Disease
- Chronic Obstructive Lung Disease
- Group Therapy Evaluation of a patient information manual

- A Social Worker in a general practice
- FACMIS, a system of keeping medical records.

The work of sending out requests to the oracles and reporting their opinions to the applicants was done by Dr. Garson, with help from his office and from his best friend and critic, his wife, Ruth. What a help it would have been if we had had the later benefits of clear and easy photocopies, fax machines, computer word-processing and E-mail!!!

Other communications

The patient records

The gold mine of information, described by Jim Collyer, could be used for retrospective studies if the records were reasonably complete. For prospective studies, details could be recorded in ways that made extraction or transfer of data accurate, but a system of checking and confirming data was advisable.

Records of patient contacts in or out of the office were especially important in group practice where several doctors might become involved with a patient over time. Even for the usual doctor, good notes served as reminders of past contacts and an advantage in assessing current problems. Dr. Wayne Weston described the gradual adoption of the problem-oriented system in his group practice, and the apparent improvement in care as a result (Weston, W.W., 1973). That might be a benefit to the practice, but not necessarily set up in a way that results could be copied and compared in other practices. For any project, the objectives must be clear, and recording consistent so that results can be useful for comparison and publication.

Patient – doctor communication

The essential for good care is the ability for both parties to listen, and to say the things necessary to identify the problems and to deal with them effectively, together.

Writing for publication

A study might have provided valuable results, of great interest and satisfaction to the researcher, but it was necessary to learn how to put all the relevant details of planning and execution into a form which was complete and concise. In the absence of word-processors, there was usually a requirement for a type-written double-spaced manuscript, with multiple copies. Each journal might have variations in its format, until the Convention of Vancouver provided a format which was accepted by most journals which we were likely to use. However, each journal publishes the advice about its own requirements, and should be consulted before anything is prepared for submission.

There are many reference books on the process of writing, the organization of data and the economy of words. Dr. Jim Collyer found that an editorial consultant could be very helpful, and advised other researchers that they would have a better chance of publication if such expert advice was obtained.

It is important for researchers to publish the results of their work whenever possible, to add to the body of family medicine. The sharing of their experience can be of benefit to others, as well as providing the opportunity of feedback to the author to confirm, challenge, or expand on the results. Even negative results are of value, both for the information obtained and perhaps to help others to avoid wasting time in doing the same thing.

Summation

The result of all research is expected to be of benefit to patients, by the process of communication. Research can find answers, but they need to be passed along so that they can be used in practice.

Chapter 7

Research Methods

The methods of doing research vary with the reason for doing it. Therefore we were impressed with the need to define our goals, by developing a question or a hypothesis. A clear question could give a clear answer, just as an ambiguous question could produce an inaccurate answer. Each word must be clearly understood, and defined if necessary. Once the question is stated clearly, the approach to an answer becomes logical. Many of the studies described above were clear and simple in their approach, and gave credible results.

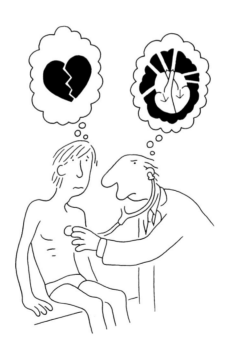

The unique opportunities in general practice were to record and study the work done in general practice by those who were doing it. Studies have often been done by observers, who were in community health or social services, but their perspective was different, even though they were skilled in their own fields. A variety of methods for organizing the records of day-to-day practice was available, to provide a cumulative description of the work done by general practitioners. Much of this recording led to specific studies of aspects of interest.

Points to consider in planning

To make best use of the time spent, it was necessary to learn the basics of planning. These were covered in the workshops and seminars described in Chapter 5, and still need to be emphasized.

- Has this question already been answered to your satisfaction? The literature search can tell you. When the Canadian Library of Family Medicine was formed by the College, in space provided by the UWO, it provided good access to family practice literature and help in literature searches.
- Which details are important? Usually, identification of the subjects of interest are necessary – name, date of birth, sex, location, and family must be considered, along with the variables of interest in the study. As in all aspects of medical contacts, confidentiality must be preserved and anyone having access to data must be aware of this need.
- Who are needed on the research team? Sometmes only one, but often it is necessary to identify the positions of principal investigator, project director, office personnel, statistician, research assistant, or recorders.
- What is the timetable? Duration of a study has a direct bearing on its cost. It must be long enough to answer the questions clearly, but not so long that the cost exceeds the limits of the granting agency.

- How will it be funded? Grant applications need to estimate pay scales, benefits, and material costs. Small grants are often available for helping to prepare an application for a larger grant.
- How will data be analyzed? Planning is necessary, and might require early consultation with a biostatistician.
- Who will write the report? Usually the principal investigator will be responsible, but will have help from some members of the team.
- What are the plans for publication? There is never a guarantee that any journal will accept it, but the intention should be to publish the results, whether positive or negative. The writing needs to be organized in the format required by the journal of choice.
- Who will be listed as authors? The journal is likely to have guidelines, limiting the names chosen to those who have made a significant contribution to the study or to an arbitrary number. In recent years, there has been wide agreement among journals about the format required.

Many of the studies mentioned in previous chapters were done before there was much help in planning. Often there was no need to make applications for grants, as the expenses involved were not great and the most important factors were the original idea and the interest of the researcher. One of the potential benefits from grant applications, besides financing, is the feedback from reviewers, who often have suggestions which might improve the study. Reviewers are usually selected because of some familiarity or experience with the topic.

In the early days, the patient was referred to as a patient. For various reasons, not necessarily valid, there has been a trend towards using the word 'client' (sociological?) or 'consumer' (political?). The euphemism 'customer' might be preferred by economists, who persist in their claim that doctors are out to maximize their income just as the rest of the population is said to be. There seems to be no recognition of a genuine goal of most physicians to do good work for their patients, with a secondary goal of earning a reasonable income. The frequent news items about doctors pushing for more fair payment have been prominent only since the government assumed control of the monopoly it created. Even before the government assumed control, it came as a surpise that to set up a practice required a business license in Victoria. Curiosity might lead to a study of the number of physicians involved in government or management roles, compared with the number forty or fifty years ago. It is probably too late to measure the thickness of carpets and the price of furniture in the executive offices for comparison with a more austere time.

However, in the interest of having an organized approach to patient care, we might think in terms of a customer who has a need, and a doctor who has the ability to meet the need. The doctor can best meet the need if armed with the right tools – mainly the knowledge of what to do and the equipment to do it with. Collectively, through research, publications and conferences, knowledge is gained and passed on for the benefit of patients and care of their problems.

For some studies, the first basic need was to know the number of patients "at risk" in a practice, with their age and sex. Age was recorded preferably as the date of birth. Other details might be relevant, such as place of residence or length of time in the practice. Sometimes place of birth or ethnicity might be relevant. With the basic information it was possible to compare with practices anywhere where similar data were recorded.

When statistics were compiled for incidence and prevalence of diseases or problems, there was a need to think in terms of equations, with a numerator and a denominator. There were several methods of describing or counting the patients in a practice, who made up the denominator, and to classify their problems to count the numerator.

The denominator

It is impossible to know exactly how many patients a doctor is responsible for, in spite of the various methods of keeping track of them. In any practice, the number of patients contacted during a year is not the same as the number at risk. Various studies have shown that anywhere from 70 to 90 percent of the population at risk might be seen in any one year. In compiling a list of patients, the question asked for each was – "if this person should have a medical problem, would I be the physician of first choice?". Many people are relatively healthy and go for years without medical attention, but are in families which have a family doctor. They know that they would call on the family doctor if necessary, and the doctor also knows it as well because of the family ties. In maintaining a practice register, all patients for whom the doctor is responsible are entered, so that the incidence of any one condition can be based on a reasonably accurate denominator of patients at risk. Casual patients can be recorded, but should be considered as separate from the practice population for purposes of estimating rates of incidence and prevalence of disease in the practice population, and in group studies.

Age-sex registers

In Britain, where patient files were presented to the general practitioner for inclusion on his list, there was a presumption that the practice registers were accurate – and perhaps they were, within the statistical variation limits. In reality, there was a delay factor when patients moved away or changed doctors. Some might not present their cards to the new doctor until there was a medical problem, and sometimes there was an administrative delay in the process of transferring medical records , often several months. Apart from delay at the government end, the capitation payment for a patient continued until his patient record folder was sent to the local council of the new doctor, at the request of the patient. To develop a patient list which was realistic, it was necessary to have a recording method which could be used to compare practices. This approach was described by Pinsent in detail, as 'The Evolving Age-sex Register' (Pinsent, R.J.F.H., 1968).

The register in the U.K. was usually kept on 3"x5" index cards, with the relevant details described above. In practices connected with the research group, up-dating the list was most important, to come as close as possible to reality.

Other practice registers

In visiting or talking to colleagues, we learned of various methods used by indviduals interested in keeping track of their patients. Medical students have often kept note books listing patient contacts. In office practice, index cards were used either to list individuals or families. In Edinburgh, Dr. Ekke Kuenssberg used a register (the F Book) similar to the E Book, having all family members listed on one page, also recording their medical encounters. (Kuennsberg, E. V., 1964). This provided a quick reference to the total family experience.

Edge-punch cards gave an easier capability for retrieving data. They had holes along the edges, each of which was labelled to show one detail about the patient, such as age-group, sex, residence, diagnoses, tests, consultations. A special punch was used to remove the outside edges of holes which were of interest. Cards were sorted with a knitting needle, which allowed punched-out sections to fall out. I think this method was used by Dr. John Fry, who has written extensively about his large practice in Beckenham, Kent. It was a fore-runner of the computer systems now in use, giving a yes-no response to each hole.

One simple method, which I used, was to have a loose-leaf book with one page per year, dating back to the oldest patient. Each page was divided vertically, with females on the right and males on the left. The day and month of birth were recorded, and the year of the entry into or exit from the practice.

This gave a permanent record which could be counted at any time. An annual count gave a picture of any trends in the practice population. The most difficult task in this or any register was to keep it current, cancelling those who had left but leaving them on the list for future reference. A general custom was to use an arbitrary time, such as two years, for deleting the name of a patient who had not been seen, unless there was a well-known family connection. [I remember well an elderly patient who had not been seen for eight years, until she turned up with a Colles fracture.] This loose-leaf system was the first introduced in Britain (Watts, C.A.H., 1963). It was replaced by the card system when there was a need to add information or to keep names in alphabetical order.

Another way of recording families is a loose-leaf book holding one page for each year from the start of the practice. As well as the primary patient (mother or father) it can list all members of the family who are considered to be patients. When counted, these numbers can give a picture of the continuity and stability in a practice. In our practice, some of the original patients were there, but the largest numbers were in the last few years.

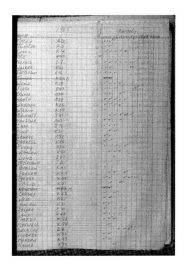

Family register

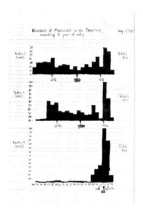

Profile shows continuity and stability. Bottom line is new member in old practice

In Canada, with no patient registration requirement, a register could be maintained only through knowledge of the patients who were apparently related to the practice. In practices with research interest the up-dating of records was done consistently, with specifically-defined criteria, and should therefore be reasonably accurate. In any system there are potential errors, but in an established practice in an area with a relatively stable population it is likely that the errors willl cancel each other out. Patients entering and leaving the practice would not change the compositon of the practice greatly, except for gradually changing with the advancing ages of the doctors and the patients.

Statistics provided by the computerized payment systems of the medical plans were of limited value.

The Numerator

Once the denominator was established as the approximate number of patients in the practice, by age and sex, it then became possible to estimate the incidence and prevalence of any diseases or other problems in the practice. These became the numerator in the equation. For realistic comparison between practices or countries, it was essential to record details in a common language.

Classifications

When Dr. Peter Postuk in Duncan, B.C., started his recording in the fifties, there was no classification suitable for general practice in Canada. His use of the Merck Manual was logical at the time, as the International Classification of Diseases (I.C.D.) was much too large and detailed but still did not include all problems seen or services provided in general practice, and the manual was readily available.

The RCGP Classification

A more practical classification was developed by the Royal College of General Practitioners, with only 365 rubrics. It included confirmed diagnoses, but provided also for signs and symptoms which might be recorded on a first visit at the highest level of certainty. The 1963 revision was included in *'A Handbook for Research in General Practice'*, edited by Eimerl and Laidlaw (Eimerl, T.S., 1969). It was also available as a 9"x9" desk-top plastic card, printed on both sides. Allowance was made for rare diseases, but the emphasis was on the common problems managed by the general practitioners. While the I.C.D. focused on diagnoses, the RCGP included morbidity, with the ability to record the diagnostic impression at each patient encounter to the highest level of certainty. For example, the most accurate diagnosis might be 'abdominal pain' recorded in the section for symptoms, rather than 'possible appendicitis' recorded in the gastro-intestinal section. A later entry might be more specific, such as duodenal ulcer or cholecystitis.

When I started recording diagnoses in 1964, the HICD Classification, adapted for hospitals, was availble (a spare copy from the Royal Jubilee Hospital in Victoria) and provided a basis for developing the routine of recording diagnoses in the E book. Later, the RCGP Classification proved to be easier to work with, although still not fully compatible with Canadian practice.

The Canuck Book

Drs. Robert Westbury and Michael Tarrant, in Calgary, Alberta, were unhappy enough with the shortcomings of the RCGP classification that they did something about it. They assembled the *'Canuck Classification'* (informally known as the Canook Book), which was more appropriate for Canadian practices (Westbury, R.C. and Tarrant, M., 1969). This was eventually used as part of the basis for the WONCA Classification, developed by an international committee chaired by Dr. Westbury.

ICHPPC

This *'International Classification of Health Problems in Primary Care'* (ICHPPC, pronounced 'Itchpick') provided a practical compromise to allow comparisons of data between countries (International, 1975).

For personal use, I found that each of the classifications could be used fairly easily, with its limitations, and that the commonest conditions comprising the majority of entries were memorized without a deliberate effort.

Prepaid medical plans

When the variety of prepaid medical insurance plans was replaced by the Medical Services Plan for B.C., it was tempting to consider the possibility of obtaining statistics from the plan, to show in detail the conditions for which patients were visiting their doctors. The plan was intended to cover all residents of B.C., and did cover the majority. The volume of data might have been of some epidemiological significance, except for several major flaws:

- the diagnosis had to be acceptable to the billing system to expedite payment, although sometimes it might not be the best description of the problem.
- multiple diagnoses could not be accommodated, even though many patients had more than one problem at any one visit.
- repeat visits would result in duplicate recording of diagnoses, whereas the object of recording was usually to show the number of patients with any diagnosis in one year. A hypertensive patient might be seen six times in a year, so the incidence of hypertension will vary greatly according to the method of recording.
- an attempt to obtain data for research purposes was rejected, because the plan's budget could not allow the extra work involved.
- the denominator, or the number of patients at risk, could not be identified, as there was no distinction betweeen regular and casual patients.

It became obvious that diagnoses submitted for the purpose of receiving payment did not always coincide with the most appropriate diagnosis or reason for attending. For example, a routine checkup was not covered by the plan, but a diagnosis of anxiety or chest pain was covered. In a similar plan in Newfoundland, where Papanicolau smears were not covered, there was a large incidence of leucorrhoea compared with B.C. where pap smears were covered and encouraged.

Diagnostic Indexes

In the early years, computers were not in common use, but it was expected that they would eventually be processing data from practice. In Britain, the most widely-used method of morbidity recording was the E Book, named after Dr. Teviot Eimerl of Liverpool, who developed it. The E Book was designed for recording and processing by hand, but was set up for computer compatibility. It was a multi-ring binder with overlapping 3"x5" pages, one for each rubric (item or diagnosis) in the RCGP Classification. Each page had ten lines on each side for recording the name and date of birth for each patient with the diagnosis for that page, with males on the front and females on the reverse. This register was a simple desk-top method of recording diagnoses, symptoms, and whatever other relevant data might be required.

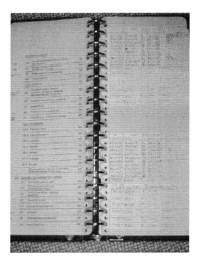

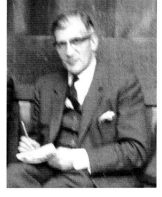

Dr. Teviot Eimerl

The E Book

In a college (RCGP) study, results were collected from over fifty widely-scattered practices, for comparison and combination. They were collated at the General Practice Research Unit in Birmingham and reported periodically in publications. These results were of enough interest to lead to the first of several National Morbidity Surveys supported by the government Department of Health and Social

Services. Apart from the contribution to group studies, the E Book was a help to the practice, with permanent and easily-found information about patients which could be a help in practice management and in recall of patients with conditions which should be followed up.

The first use of the E Book in Canada was in Newfoundland, where Dr. John Ross of St. John's and Dr. Mel Parsons of Glovertown took part in the Transatlantic Morbidity Survey along with British recorders (Transatlantic, 1969). At the meeting of WONCA in Montreal in 1964, when Dr. Robin Pinsent demonstrated the E Book, Dr. Jim Fowler of Victoria, B.C., showed enough interest that a copy was sent to him. He was not ready to start recording, so I was able to take his book and start to record all patient contacts. Entries were made at the time of a visit, or by an assistant using the daily list of patients and diagnoses. The early experience in 1964-65 was a great help when I visited Dr. Pinsent and the Birmingham Research Unit of the RCGP, as I could better understand the work of the recorders and see the value of their accumulated data.

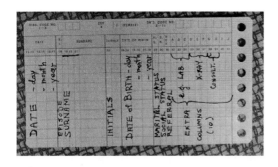

Details of
Recording on
E Book page

Once entries were made into the E Book, data could be extracted easily, quickly, and cheaply. If you wondered how many patients you had with any condition, such as hypertension, pregnancy or arthritis, you could turn to the appropriate page for an immediate count. If you recorded follow-up visits, you could also see the number of visits or the outcomes of treatment for each condition. Whereas the prepaid medical plans, as a rule, could enter only one diagnosis per billing card, the E Book could record all diagnoses which were treated or discussed at each visit.The E Book was used in other countries. In Australia, the journal *'Annals of General Practice'* donated fifty to the Australian College of General Practitioners, and by 1965 there were 26 in use. In New Zealand at that time there were about fifty in use. The books were available in Canada through the College office, and soon there were 66 reported in B.C. and many in other provinces.

The F Book was in a format similar to the E Book, but provided for the recording of encounters for all members of a family on one page. Dr. Ekke Kuenssberg, of Edinburgh, developed this method of giving a comprehensive picture of the family health and patterns of illness, which sometimes were from non-infectious causes such as coronary disease, ulcers, or psychiatric problems (Kuenssberg, E.V., 1964).

Specific lists

For their own interest, some doctors have kept lists of patients whom they considered to be of most significance in terms of followup. The usual problems of hypertension, diabetes, headaches or arthritis could be recorded easily on plain paper or in a format such as the E book. There could be as many other problems listed as were considered appropriate, including such items as poverty, single parents, child behavior, accidents or violence – the list could be long.

Questionnaires

Production of a good questionnaire is a form of art. It sometimes seemed that questionnaires we received in the practice were prepared rather quickly – perhaps dictated but not read. Any group wanting information would feel comfortable compiling and sending one out without consultation with the research committee. Even if the first draft was perfect, there was still the possibility that some would benefit from advice, and also the research committee would benefit from the exercise of reviewing and considering whether it could be improved.

In the early years and later, it became important to recognize the difficulty in preparing a questionnaire and to keep in mind the main principles:

- Clarity – there must be no ambiguity; each word must have only one possible meaning.
- Language – plain words, with definitions of any which might be unfamiliar to some of the respondents.
- Economy – only the items really needed should be included; the temptation to add extras which are unlikely to help in the study must be controlled.
- Completeness – all the needed elements should be included, as there might not be another chance to ask.
- Testing – to achieve accurate results, a questionnaire should first be tried on a small sample of friends or colleagues who will not be subjects in the study; this testing might need to be repeated several times, as problems are identified.
- Format – a combination of eye appeal and simplicity will help the responder to find time to complete the questionnaire.
- Computer compatibility – sometimes spacing and arrangements can be set up for the convenience of the data processor – a worthy objective if it does not also make the form less attractive to the eye and not so easy to complete.
- Significance - not least, the purpose of the questionnaire must make sense to those who are expected to complete it.

The problem of quality in construction of questionnaires was highlighted by Dr. Don Farquhar, who reacted to a poorly-designed request for information about original package dispensing. He was upset enough to write a letter to the Canadian Family Physician (Farquhar, D., 1971).

Statistics

The worst way to get help from a statistician was to do a study and then ask to have the statistical analysis done. Advice from individuals and from various workshops emphasized the need to include the statistical factors at an early stage of planning. The usual medical school and residency training did not include much teaching in statistics, so either the prospective researcher had to learn enough to use in the project or ask for expert consultation, preferably with a biostatistician.

Among the many texts available was the highly-regarded book by Sir Austin Bradford Hill, which was (and is) readable and logical (Hill, A.B., 1961).

Ideally, at least one pilot study would be done to test the method and the plan for analysis of data. The pilot would help to determine sample size and the details for recording data. Too large a sample is wasteful of time and money, while too small a sample is also wasteful of time and money because it will not produce significant results. For economy, it was necessary to focus on the details of importance, and avoid the temptation to add extra items. In an extreme and unusual happening, one case could be significant if a previously incurable disease was cured.

The RCGP recognized the importance of expert advice by including a statistican, Ken Cross, in the research unit at Birmingham,.

Most important, it was necessary to understand the meaning of relevant terms - especially incidence, prevalence, rates of morbidity and mortality, rubric, cohort, case-control, randomization.

To maintain confidentiality, a simple method was devised by Hogben, a mathematician. If the first three letters of the surname, the first initial and the date of birth (HOGJ 251259) are recorded, these ten digits are unlikely to be duplicated within a population of 50 million, except for identical twins.

Summary card

The Summary Card is a useful way of condensing records to make them more readily available, especially with thick charts. The card below is based on the one developed by Dr. Ashley Aitkin, in Oamaru, New Zealand, as mentioned on page 16. This example is from my own practice. The time taken to summarize might be saved from time needed in leafing through multiple pages of assorted records.

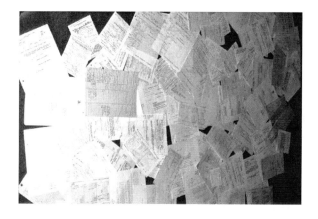

Old reports (above) replaced by the new Summary Card (right)

Ethics

Consideration of research methods would be incomplete without a reminder of the need to be aware of possible ethical problems. In all research, the principle of confidentiality must be observed. Reports of results must preserve patient privacy, by omitting names or identifying features.

When patients are involved in clinical or therapeutic trials, informed consent must be obtained. They should be told the reasons for the project, the risks, the random allocation, and the possible benefits to them or to mankind. They should also be informed that they can quit at any time without prejudice. One problem in assuring informed consent is the difficulty of knowing that a patient understands all the details, and has read what is sometimes a lengthy or legalistic document.

An early example of the difficulty in achieving confidentiality was provided by a patient of mine. She had quit working for the provincial medicare plan. She could not tolerate the gossip among the clerks, who recognized friends or well-known people in the claims.

At the suggestion of Dr. John Garson, the National Research Committee of the College was among the first in Canada to acknowledge the importance of the Declaration of Helsinki, and require its application in any research proposals (Falk,W.A., Research Newspage, 1974). The declaration was short and simple, aimed at protection of the patient from the possible hazards of research.

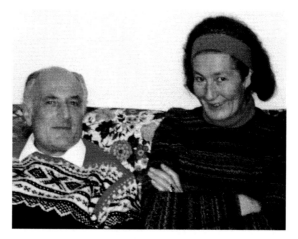

Dr. John Z. and Ruth (Curly) Garson

Chapter 8

Finances

Even family doctors need to earn a living. In private general practice there was no university or public health salary to compensate the principal investigator for time spent on research. Grants were available to help with the costs of materials and a research assistant or director, but nothing to pay for the time of the doctor who is responsible for the project. Unless this policy has changed recently, lack of income is still a deterrent to heavy involvement in a project. One general practitioner in Hobart, Tasmania, Dr. Paul Clark, had an idea for a laboratory test for cancer which turned out to be more expensive than he had anticipated. He was relieved when the pilot project failed, as he would have been morally obliged to continue if results had been positive (Clark, P.S., 1964).

In spite of the deficiencies in support, help was available from a variety of sources.

Personal

When the early researchers had ideas, they usually pursued their interests with the resources at hand, without applying for grants. They were compelled to satisfy their curiosity, perhaps without any training or experience. Some of the results, described in Chapter 1, were of interest and value. One of Dr. Robin Pinsent's sayings was "if you can't finance a study with money stolen from the household budget, perhaps it isn't worth doing". This concept might not be popular in the household, but he makes a good point - that information of value can be obtained with relatively little cost, and possibly using less time than would be needed to prepare a grant application and to wait for a response. Examples of simple but useful studies were mentioned earlier, such as Dr. W.O. Williams' method of recording flu patients on a roll of paper and Dr. Will Pickles' records of infectious disease in his isolated practice.

Entering into the E Book did not take much time or training. Help was willingly given by our daughter Andrea (in high school) at the cost of one penny per line. [She has become a Macintosh expert, using it for a variety of activities, including translating books on Martial Arts from Chinese to English.] Results for my E Book project of recording for two years were analyzed by a computer program written by our high school son Bruce, who has become a computer programmer.

The Practice

In solo practice, research might be regarded as a hobby or as an imperative when a doctor realizes that we have much to learn and a unique opportunity in general practice. The time spent is the responsibility of the individual.

In group or partnership practice each member should contribute fairly to the practice, or have partners who are willing to allow the time and disruptions involved. Even when time is granted, there might still be criticism, not always overt, if the researcher has a much lower practice volume. If there is an equal sharing of income, the researcher might be seen to contribute less than his share of the paid work. The acceptance by the outside world of the published results could be less appreciated by those who feel they have carried too much of the practice workload. One example of cooperation was in the Saskatoon Community Clinic, where Dr. John Garson was the Director of Research and had some time allotted for the research, which was considered to be of value to the clinic. In my own practice, my partners and the staff went along with my enthusiam and worked with the changes in our record system.

Private Donors

An occasional source of support was the individual patient who might wish to help because of good experience with family doctors, or simply wish to help improve general practice. Examples in the B.C. Chapter of the College included the Ethel Wallace Fund, named after a patient who left money for research to be allocated at the discretion of her family doctor, Ian Balmer. Similarly, the Lydia Foster Fund was created by a bequest from a patient of mine who had so many relatives that her estate would not provide much for anyone. She asked my advice about charities, and was presented with a variety of alternatives. As she had arthritis and hypertension among her problems, their societies were mentioned, along with the research needs of the College. After a career in nursing, she apparently thought that research by family doctors would be useful, as she bequeathed the proceeds from selling her small house to the B.C. Chapter of the College, for supporting research. A detail in the latter fund illustrated the importance of checking details. By the time the will had been probated and the lawyer had informed the College, the name by which the patient was known, Helen Forster, had been changed to Lydia Foster.

Another major bequest was provided by Dr. Douglas Robb, who had been the active New Brunswick member of the National Research Committee formed by Jim Collyer. Doug made a provision in his will which was used to establish the Douglas Robb Fund, with an annual grant available for supporting research projects by College members. This fund might still be enlarged by donations and bequests from other members of the College or the public.

The College

In the early years, there was never enough money to support all of the potential activities of the College. As the primary emphasis of the College was on education, the only significant support for research projects was provided to the College by the Mead Johnson annual grant of $5,000. However, when Dr. Jim Collyer came to the board with his well-organized plan to develop a truly national committee of members with a significant interest in research, he was given excellent support. This provided for the series of national workshops which stimulated activity across the country. It seems that the investment at that time has paid good returns, when we see the large output of research in recent years.

Attendance at the workshops by board members of the College and by Dr. Don Rice, the Executive Director, increased their awareness of the progress made, and helped them to justify the financing of efforts to establish a centre for research at the College offices.

Government

The Department of National Health and Welfare was receptive to applications for some smaller projects by individual general practitioners. Most applicants lacked credibility because of the scant history of successful projects by them or by other general practitioners.

As one way to provide training, the department of National Health and Welfare made a special effort to involve family physicians in their series of National Health Grant Seminars described earlier.

The 1973 seminar was organized by Dr. John Last in Ottawa. With the theme of Family Medicine Research, and payment for expenses of travel and accommodation, it attracted enough family physicians in a cold January to influence later progress. This seminar led to Department approval of an application by the College to hold a seminar in Victoria, in a warm November in 1975, with family doctors as the main participants (Appendix 3). The names of many of those who attended these seminars have appeared often in subsequent research projects, publications, and conferences.

Another example of a major project supported by a National Health Grant was the Nova Scotia Fetal Morbidity project. This involved Dr. Michael Hebb of Dartmouth almost fulltime for two years as a paid project director. Most of the general practitioners in Nova Scotia enrolled in this evaluation of an antenatal risk scoring system, to show its potential to reduce perinatal morbidity (Hebb, M., 1980). It happened that fetal morbidity improved, even among the practitioners who were not enrolled in the project.

Provincial and municipal departments of health or epidemiology were also capable of supporting projects. For example, I received a small National Health Grant in 1970 to pay for a part-time research assistant to process the age-sex register and E Book data for our group practice and four others in B.C. It was administered by the provincial Department of Health which had approved the application as being relevant.

Non-governmental agencies

Support has been given for various projects by other agencies such as the Vancouver Foundation, the B.C. MSI Foundation and the Alberta MSI Foundation. Dr. Kerr White, Medical Director of the Rockefeller Foundation, has been a strong supporter of NAPCRG from its beginning, and showed great interest in primary care even before that.

Business and Industry

The Mead Johnson Company, mentioned above, for ten years until 1972 provided an annual grant of $5,000 to the College without strings attached. The College board of directors, in its wisdom, decided to use the money to help with the planning and execution of small studies of interest to recipients, who were selected by the College research committee. Other companies dealt directly with individual doctors, most often in relation to evaluation of products of interest to the companies. These were group studies, in which selected practices across the country might contribute data, following the protocol set by the company paying the costs. These studies were often to monitor new drugs for previously unknown side-effects.

The value of assessment of approved drugs by general practitioners was recognized by the PMAC (Pharmaceutical Manufacturers Association of Canada) in 1959, when it approached the research committee of the College. The medical directors of companies which had worked with general practitioners had found that "important differences in opinion regarding drugs are registered by general practitioners as opposed to those physicians in the larger research centres". As general practitioners were responsible for assessment and treatment of over 80% of problems encountered by their patients, the best use of available drugs was an important part of their work. It was a natural combination to work with drug companies to assess their products in practice. The fact that costs were paid and that there were some perks was criticized. As Dr. Jim Collyer said, in 1973, "...we can do scientifically-controlled studies on large groups of patients, to truly test the drugs we use every day. Such trials are not easy, but of any group in medicine we are in the best position to do them. We see illness at an earlier stage than any other branch of medicine. We are the only ones who can tell what drugs are best for those illnesses".

The early study of the work of the general practitioner, by Clute, was made possible by grants from the Rockefeller Foundation, the Canadian Life Insurance Officers Association, and the federal Department of Health and Welfare.

Immeasurable and often unrecognized costs

The family, apart from 'money stolen from the household budget', has given moral and practical support. Often they have helped to record details or to criticize manuscripts. The interest provided by research was balanced against the time away from family required by the researcher. Occasionally, travel to meetings could include one or more family members, with a chance to learn more about other countries or other parts of Canada. Whatever the costs, for me the involvement in research has been a life-changing and enriching experience for which I am grateful.

Afterword

One of the statements often made in interviews of people who have come into the public eye is "If I had my life to live over again I wouldn't change a thing". In looking back, I can see many things I would change.

I would happily accept any suggestions for addition to this memoir, which is intended to honour pioneers who preceded the organized system we now have in The College and the universities.

In spite of the progress in our national research efforts, it has been surprising in the year 2000 to see articles written by family medicine research workers in Canada and in Britain bemoaning the lack of interest in research by family doctors. Perhaps the supposed lack of interest is real. The current pressures imposed by the shortage of family doctors and by their greater workload may leave little time or energy for research. Private practitioners might contribute to studies originating in the family medicine departments, but they are less likely to initiate studies of their own.

Yes, I joined the university Department of Family Medicine in Calgary, but sometimes I wonder whether I might have made a better contribution to research from private practice.

I trust that there will always be curious family doctors who will remain at the grass roots.

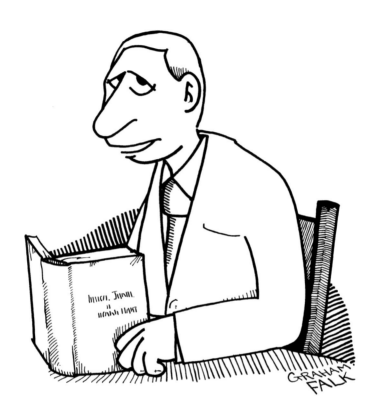

"I don't like the looks of this appendix."

Appendix 1

College of Family Physicians of Canada
National Research Conference

London, Ontario, January 17 and 18th, 1969

Support of the following is gratefully acknowledged:
  The College of Family Physicians of Canada, and chapters
of Ontario, Alberta, Manitoba, Newfoundland, British
Columbia and Saskatchewan.
  The Mead Johnson Company
  Charles E. Frosst Company of Canada Ltd
  The Elliot Cerini Foundation
  Universities of Western Ontario (Dean D. Bocking), Calgary
(Dean W. Cochrane), McMaster (Dean John Evans), Ottawa
(Dean J. Lussier) and B.C. (Dean John McCreary).

Program

Thursday, January 16: 8:00 p.m. - Reception at Holiday Inn
  8:30 - Welcome by Dean Douglas Bocking at Medical
       Sciences Building.
  Greetings from the College of Family Physicians of Canada.

Friday, January 17:
  8:45 - <u>Research and the Family Physician.</u> Prof. Ian
McWhinney, Head of Sub-dept. of Family Medicine, UWO
  9:30 - <u>Family Practice Research Throughout the World.</u>
Dr. William Falk, Nuffield Travelling Fellow, 1965.
  10:00 - <u>Our Task at this Meeting.</u> Dr. James Collyer,
Chairman, National Research Committee; conference organizer.
  11:00 - <u>Group discussions</u> - Aims of National Research
Committee.
  12:00 - <u>Plenary Session</u> - Finalize aims.
       Chairman, Dr. J. Collyer.
  1:30 - 5:00 p.m. <u>Group discussions</u>.
  6:30 - Reception and dinner at University Club.
     Speakers: Dr. Ian Watson - "New Delhi and Research".
            Dr. Donald Rice - "Recent Impressions of
       Russia and New Delhi"

121

Saturday, January 18:
>8:30 - 12:00   Plenary Sessions: Chairman, Dr. Jim Collyer.
>1:00   National Research Committee
>>Conclusions, Constitutional and Research:
>>Dr. Paul Stein, member of Nucleus Committee.
>
>2:30   Summary and Charge: Dr. Ian Watson.

Delegates

College of Family Physicians:
>Dr. Stephen Clark, President
>Dr. Donald Rice, Executive Director
>Dr. John Zack, Chairman, Coordinating Committee on Education

Central Nucleus Committee, London, Ontario:
>Drs. James A. Collyer, Cam Lamont, Jack Orchard, Keith Gay, and Paul Stein.

Provincial chapters:
>B.C. - William Falk, Victoria; John Sumner, Haney
>Alberta - Grant Mills and Robert Westbury, Calgary; Brian Du Heame, Edmonton
>Saskatchewan - Alan Clews and John Garson, Saskatoon.
>Manitoba - Hugh Fairley, St. Vital; H. Dirks, Winnipeg.
>Ontario - Alan MacFarlane, Hamilton; David Lawee, Toronto.
>Quebec - A. Burton, Mount Royal.
>New Brunswick - Arthur van Wart, Frederickton; M. Nixon, St. John.
>Prince Edward Island - Stewart MacDonald, Charlottetown.
>Nova Scotia - Iain MacPherson, Halifax; Eugene Nurse, Dartmouth.
>Newfoundland - John Ross, Placentia; Mel Parsons, Glovertown.

Guests
>Mrs. Beatrice Robinow, McMaster Biochemical Library.
>Miss Anne Schoult, Health Sciences, UWO.

Observers
>From London, Ontario:
>>Dr. A.T. Hunter, Assist. Prof. Sub-dept. of Family Medicine.
>>Dr. Glen Pratt, Chief of Family Practice, Victoria Hospital.
>>Dr. Carol Buck, Prof. and Chairman, Dept. of Community Medicine.

Dr. Charles Rand, Assoc. Prof., Epidemiology and
Preventive Medicine.

Dr. K. Stavraky, Assist. Prof., Epidemiology &
Preventive Medicine

Dr. Jack Thurlow, Counsellor, Student Health Services.

Dr. J.H. Watson, Clin. Assist. Prof., Epidemiology &
Preventive Med.

Dr. Jim Wanklin, Ph. D., Dept. of Community Medicine.

Dr. Harold Steward, Prof. of Biochem., UWO, , MRC Rep.

Dr. J. Paul Newell, 3rd. year resident, St. Joseph's Hosp.

Dr. Bill Martin, 2nd year resident, St. Joseph's Hosp.

Dr. Peter MacLoughlin, 2nd year resident, St. Joseph's
Hosp.

Dr. John Sangster, 2nd year resident, St. Joseph's Hosp.

Mr. B.P. O'Connell, Dept. of Family Medicine, McMaster
Univ. Clinic.

From Ottawa, Ontario:

Dr. Peter Heaton, Family Practice Unit.

Dr. D.W. Menzies, Director, Field Study Unit, Epidem. Div.,
D.N.H. & W.

Dr. D.F. Marcellus, Principal Medical Officer, D.N.H. & W.

From Toronto, Ontario:

Dr. Stanley Lang, Research and Planning Div. (R. & P.),
Dept. of Health.

Dr. A. Kapos, Psychologist, R. & P. Div., Dept. of Health

Dr. J.E. Knapp , Medical Director, Mead Johnson of Canada.

Mr. Dean Irwin, Medical Post

From elsewhere:

Dr. John Davies, Div. of Family Medicine, Miami, Florida.

Dr. Lee Blanchard, San Jose, California.

Dr. Henry Kedworth, Assoc. Prof., Memorial Univ.,
Newfoundland

Appendix 2

National workshops of the College of Family Physicians of Canada

1. Muskoka, Ontario, September 1970

The Muskoka Workshop, at the Sherwood Inn on Muskoka Lake, provided a great stimulus to those attending, many of whom have appeared in subsequent studies and reports. Guest faculty consisted of major contributors to the research work of the Royal College of General Practitioners (RCGP):

Dr. Donald L. Crombie, Director of the General Practice Research Unit to Council of the RCGP.

Dr. Robin J.F.H. Pinsent, Research Advisor, Research Committee to Council of the RCGP.

Dr. Ekke V. Kuenssberg, Treasurer and Secretary, Research Foundation Board to Council of the RCGP.

Dr. Clifford Kay, Recorder, Oral Contraceptive Study of Council of the RCGP.

Dr. Ian McWhinney, Head of the Division of Family Medicine at the University of Western Ontario.

Sponsors were Mead Johnson of Canada Limited, the Elliot Cerini Foundation, and The College.

Dr. Jim Collyer, the Chairman, opened the workshop with an outline of the objectives and format, followed by formal greetings from the College president, Dr. David Brunet, of Grandmere, Quebec.

Introductory talks were then given by committee members:

"The Potential of Family Practice Research", by Dr. John Z. Garson, Co-chairman, Saskatchewan Research Committee.

"Research Submission Format", by Dr. Bill Falk, Vice-chairman, National Research Committee.

"Design of Projects", by Professor Ian McWhinney.

"Problems of Disease Classification", by Dr. Robert Westbury, Chairman, Library Committee of the CFPC.

Major themes were introduced by guest faculty:
"Clinical Studies in General Practice", by Dr. Donald Crombie.
"Epidemiology in Family Practice", by Dr. Robin Pinsent.
"Organizational Studies in Practice", by Dr. Ekke Kuenssberg.
"Group Studies in Family Practice", by Dr. Clifford Kay.

After each theme was introduced, small groups met to discuss the topic and consider planning of a project, with a recorder to report results when the full group reassembled.

Delegates

included College members from across Canada:
Dr. Jim Collyer, chairman and conference coordinator
Drs. A.M. Hebb and Iain G. MacPherson – Nova Scotia
Drs. W.R. Gillis and M. Keeting - New Brunswick
Dr. A.S. MacDonald - Prince Edward Island
Drs. M.E. McDonald and Mel Parsons - Newfoundland.
Drs. Dan Glick, C. Forgiel, Peter Heaton, John
    Hilditch, Alan McFarlane, B. Riddle, and Laurie
    Zeilig - Ontario.
Drs. W.J. Blight, Henry Dirks, and J.C. Menzies -
    Manitoba.
Drs. Alan Clews, John Garson, and David Road –
    Saskatchewan.
Drs. Howard Gretton, Claude Labelle, Michael
    Tarrant, Robert Westbury, D.J. Wharton - Alberta.
Drs. Brian Allen, Brian Dixon-Warren, Bill Falk,
    Dennis Moore, and John Sumner – British Columbia

Details are listed because of the importance of the Muskoka workshop as a major step in the development of an enthusiastic group in Canada, many of whom have contributed to family medicine research and teaching.

2. Banff, Alberta, Sept. 17-18, 1971

The workshop at the Timberline Hotel was organized by Drs. Michael Tarrant and Robert Westbury of Calgary, to precede the annual scientific session of the College and to follow a meeting of the National Research Committee.

Guest Faculty were:
Dr. Harding Le Riche, Professor and Chairman of the Department of Epidemiology and Biometrics, U. Of Toronto (under whom Dr. John Garson later studied for the Diploma in Epidemiology and Community Health).

Dr. Edgar J. Love, Professor of Community Health Science, U. of Calgary.

Dr. James M. Wanklin, Associate Professor, Department of Community Medicine, U.W.O.

Dr. Donald C. Ferguson, Ph.D., Assistant Professor of International Health, School of Hygiene and Public Health, Johns Hopkins University in Baltimore, Maryland.

Program

Techniques in finding, recording and analyzing information for research in family practice.

Friday, September 17
1. Practical problems of research in our offices
    (i) Group Morbidity/Epidemiological Studies:
        a) Newfoundland/Great Britain 1969 study
            Dr. Mel Parsons, Glovertown South, NF.
        b) B.C. - 56 Practice Study
            Dr. Bill Falk, Victoria, B.C.
        c) Comments – Dr. John Sumner, Maple
        Ridge, B.C.
    (ii) Clinical Studies - Measuring Treatment:
        a) Treatment of sore throats
            Dr. Al MacFarlane, Hamilton, Ont.
        b) Treatment of emotional illness
            Dr. David Road, Regina, Sask.
        c) Comments – Dr. John Garson, Saskatoon,
    (iii) Group Study Problems:
        a) How we found 170 participants
            Dr. Iain MacPherson, Halifax, N.S.

b) High risk pregnancy problems
   Dr. Michael Hebb, Dartmouth, NS
c) Comments – Dr. Alan Clews, Saskatoon, SK.
(iv) Basis of a family practice record keeping system. Committee report – Dr. Grant Mills, Edmonton, AB

2. Immeasurables:
   (i) How to measure the art of medicine
        Chairman – Dr. Donald Ferguson
        a) Discussion
        b) Work sessions, small groups
        c) Reporting session

Saturday, September 18
1. Designing studies:
   (i) How many, how much, how long? - James Wanklin, Ph.D.
        a) Work Sessions, small groups
        b) Reporting session
   (ii) How to keep track - Dr. Harding leRiche
        a) Work sessions, small groups
        b) Reporting session

Sunday, September 19
1. What does it mean? – Dr. Edgar Love, Calgary, AB
        a) Work sessions, small groups
        b) Reporting sessions
2. Summary – Dr. Robert Westbury, Calgary, AB

Among those also present were Drs. Stan Sinclair (Montreal. P.Q.), Brian Fern (Saskatoon, SK), Henry Dirks (Winnipeg, Man.), Brian Dixon-Warren (Meadow Lake, SK). The complete list is missing so far.

3. Chester, Nova Scotia Workshop, May 1972

The session at the Longboat Inn was organized by Dr. Iain MacPherson and his committee. Unlike the workshops in 1970 and 1971, most of the talks and discussions were conducted by the family medicine research committee of the College. Like the others, its expenses were met by The College.

Aim: To provide a basic training in family practice research

Faculty: members of National Research Committee

      Dr. Bill Falk, Victoria, B.C.

      Dr. Robert Westbury, Calgary, AB

      Dr. John Garson, Saskatoon, SK

      Dr. Iain MacPherson, Halifax, NS

Small group chairmen:

      Dr. Mel Parsons, Glovertown South, NF

      Dr. Mike Hebb, Dartmouth, NS

      Dr. David Road, Regina, SK

      Dr. Stanley Sinclair, Montreal, PQ

Monday, May 29

1. Family practice as a source of research:

      Studies – Defining your aims. What interests you in practice?

      a) Dr. John Garson

      b) Small groups

      c) Reporting session

2. Design of projects:

      Basic principles: How to measure your interest.

      a) Dr. Robert Westbury

      b) Small groups

      c) Reporting session

Tuesday, May 30

1. Group projects:

      a) Dr. Iain MacPherson

      b) Small groups

      c) Reporting session

2. Reporting methods available: E Books, specific forms, computers – pros and cons
                a) Dr. Bill Falk
                b) Small groups
                c) Reporting session
3. Summary of the two days: Dr. Alan Clews.

Both evenings: Informal programs –
      Use of the Spoken and Written Word
              Miss Ursula Matthews, editorial consultant
              Mr. John Duckworth, actor and director

The complete list of those attending the workshop has not yet been found. However, we can remember the presence of Dr. Donald Rice, who has attended most of the research committee meetings. During a break, he drove several of us to see his hometown of Bridgewater, a beautiful area near Lunenberg. We also remember the enthusiastic presence of Drs. Maurice Wood and Jack Froom, who had just attended the first meeting of NAPCRG, in Richmond,VA. It was the start of great progress in the U.S.A., which was helped by the support of Dr. Kerr White.

Appendix 3

The National Health Grant Seminar on Research in Family Medicine, University of Ottawa, February 4-9, 1973

List of family physicians attending

Dr. Richard Bann - Ottawa, Ontario - Family Physician, Director of Clinic

Dr. Gary Beazley - Winnipeg, Family Physician

Dr. Douglas Black - Baie Verte, Newfoundland – Medical Superintendent and Family Physician

Dr. Louis Christ - Saskatoon - Head of Family Medicine, U. of Saskatchewan

Dr. Gordon Dickie - London, Ontario - Family Medicine Centre

Dr. Henry Dirks - Winnipeg

Dr. Bill Falk - Victoria, B.C. - Chairman, National Research Committee of the College

Dr. Michael Hebb - Dartmouth, Nova Scotia - Coordinator,

Dr. David Lawee – Toronto

Dr. George McQuitty – Calgary - Dept. of Family Medicine, U. of Calgary

Dr. Wyn Rhys-Jones - Ottawa, Ontario

Dr. Walter Rosser - Ottawa, Ontario

Dr. Jim Wilson - London, Ontario

List of Tutors

Dr. John Cassell - Physician Epidemiologist, Professor and Chairman, Dept. of Epidemiology, School of Public Health, U. of North Carolina

Dr. Donald L. Crombie - General Practitioner, Birmingham, England; Visiting Professor, Dept. of Family Medicine, UWO; Chairman of Research Committee, Royal College of General Practitioners.

Dr. John Fry - General Practitioner, Beckenham, Kent, England; elder statesman in Royal College of General Practitioners and author of books on general practice

Dr. Keith Hodgkin - General Practitioner in Redcar, Yorkshire; recently Visiting Professor at Memorial University, St. John's, Newfoundland, in Dept. of Family Medicine

Dr. Arthur Kraus - Statistician, Associate Professor, Dept. of Community Health and Epidemiology, Queen's University, Kingston, Ontario

Dr. John Last - Physician Epidemiologist, Professor and Chairman, Department of Epidemiology and Community Medicine, U. of Ottawa

Dr. Edward Love - Statistician, Medical Educator, Acting Head, Division of Community Health Sciences, U. of Calgary

Dr. Ian McWhinney - Family Physician Educator, Professor and Chairman, Dept. of Family Medicine, U. of Western Ontario

Dr. R. John C. Pearson - Physician Epidemiologist, Associate Professor, Dept. of Epidemiology and Community Medicine, U., of Ottawa

Dr. David L. Sackett - Internist Epidemiologist, Professor and Chairman, Dept. of Clinical Epidemiology and Biostatistics, McMaster U., Hamilton, Ontario

Dr. Walter O. Spitzer - Family Physician, Epidemiologist, Associate Professor of Clinical Epidemiology and Biostatistics, and of Family Medicine, McMaster U., Hamilton, Ontario

List of Consultants

Thomas J. Boudreau - Economist, Dept. of Behavioural Sciences, University of Sherbrooke

Darlene Flett - Public Health Nurse Epidemiologist, Dept. of Epidemiology and Community Medicine, U. of Ottawa

Lorie Marrett - Statistician, Dept. of Epidemiology and Community Medicine, U. of Ottawa

Jan Pool - Social Survey Research Worker, Dept. of Epidemiology and Community medicine, U. of Ottawa

Pamela Poole - Nursing Consultant, National Health and Welfare, Ottawa

S. Raman - Statistician, Dept. of Epidemiology annd Community Medicine, U. of Ottawa

Stephen Walter - Statistician, Dept. of Epidemiology and Community Medicine, U. of Ottawa

John Western - Anthropologist, Visiting Professor in the Dept. of Epidemiology and Community Medicine, U. of Ottawa, from Australia

Appendix 4

The National Health Grant Seminar on Research in Family Medicine, held in
Victoria, B.C., November 9-14, 1975

Students, included seventeen general practitioners/family doctors. Another seven were from the disciplines of Social Work, Nursing, and Psychology. The family doctors were at various levels of practice, from one in a residency, some in private practice or clinics, and others in university teaching programs. Their experience in research ranged from very little to extensive. Those in family medicine were:

Dr. William Bryant, Kitchener, Ontario.
Dr. Alex Cherkezoff, Vancouver, B.C.
Dr. James Collyer, London, Ontario.
 Dr. F. Dean Collett, Medical Director, Inglewood Health Centre,
          Calgary, Alberta.
Dr. Paul Duchastel, Centre Medical, St. Bruno, Quebec.
Dr. Wayne Elford, Assistant Professor, Division of Family Practice,
          University of Calgary, Alberta.
Dr. Richard Hibbard, Saskatoon Community Clinic, Saskatchewan.
Dr. Michael Johnston, Moncton Medical Clinic, Moncton, N.B.
Dr. Craig Karpilow, Resident in Family Practice,
          Memorial University, St. John's, Newfoundland.
Dr. Sydney Librach, Family Practice and Teaching, University of
          Toronto, Western Hospital.
Dr. Robert J. McBride, Medical Consultant, Medical Programs
          Branch, Ontario Ministry of Health.
Dr. Jacqueline McClaren, Hertzl Family Practice Centre, McGill
          University, Montreal, Quebec.
Dr. R. Wayne Putnam, Assistant Director, Division of Continuing
          Education, Dalhousie University, Halifax, N.S.
Dr. Linda Rapson, Acupuncture Foundation of Canada, Toronto.
Dr. Michael Tarrant, Cambrian Clinic, Calgary, Alberta.
Dr. V. Jim Thorsteinson, Clinical Demonstrator in Family Practice,
          University of Manitoba, Winnipeg.
Dr. Robert Westbury, Cambrian Clinic, Calgary, Alberta.

Tutors for this ninth seminar in the series were:

Dr. Carol Buck, Professor of Epidemiology & Preventive Medicine at U.W.O.

Robert G. Evans, Ph.D., Associate Professor, Dept. of Economics at U.B.C.

Dr. William A. Falk, Family Physician, Victoria, B.C.

Brenda Fraser, Ph.D., Assistant Professor, Department of Health Care & Epidemiology, U.B.C.

Dr, John Z. Garson, Family Physician, Clinical Coordinator, Community Clinic, Saskatoon, Saskatchewan.

Dr. Keith Hodgkin, Professor and Chairman, Department of General Practice, Memorial University, St. John's, Newfoundland.

John Horne, Ph.D., Assistant Professor, Department of Social & Preventive Medicine, University of Manitoba.

Dr. Edgar J. Love, Professor, Division of Community Health Sciences, University of Calgary, Alberta.

Dr. Alexander MacPherson, Chief, Department of Community Health, Montreal General Hospital.

Pamela E. Poole, R.N., Chief, Information & Evaluation Division, Research Programs Directorate, Department of Health & Welfare, Ottawa.

Dr. David L. Sackett, Professor of Clinical Epidemiology, Biostatistics & Medicine, McMaster University Medical Centre, Hamilton, Ontario.

Dr. Robert A. Spasoff, Associate Professor of Community Health & Epidemiology, Queen's University, Kingston, Ontario.

Morton Warner, PG Diploma in Applied Social Studies, Assistant Professor and Chairman, Division of Health Services Planning, U.B.C.

Consultants who were available on request included:

Charles A. Laszlo, Ph.D., Associate Director, Division of Health Systems, U.B.C.

Charles Aharan, Ph.D., Program Director, Victoria Life Enrichment Society.

Martin Collis, Ph.D., Associate Professor, Department of Physical Education, University of Victoria.

Leonard Hole, M.P.H., Research Supervisor, Division of Vital Statistics, Community Health Programs Division, Victoria.

Thomas Maguire, Ph.D., Professor and Chairman, Division of Psychological Foundations in Education, U. of Victoria.

Jack Rowe, M.P.H., Biostatistician, Division of Vital Statistics, Community Health Programs Division, Victoria.

Glossary

ACGP = The Australian College of General Practitioners

CFPC or The College = The College of Family Physicians of Canada (from 1967).

CGP = The College of General Practitioners (Britain, up to 1962)

CGPC = The College of General Practice of Canada (up to 1967).

Curious = 1. Eager to learn; inquisitive. 2. Interesting because of oddness or novelty; strange; unexpected (Collins, 1983).

Denominator = the number of patients in the group under study;
or the patients "at risk" in a practice.

Family Medicine = the body of knowledge for teaching, research and the provision of primary medical care.

General practice = the conduct of general medical practice or family practice, or the office or centre where such work is done.

G.P./F.P. = the terms "general practitioner" and "family physician" were used interchangeably, the former in Britain, Australia, and New Zealand (and many other countries), the latter in Canada and the U.S.A.

ICHPPC = The International Classification of Health Problems
in Primary Care (for convenience, pronounced as Itchpic).

IEA = International Epidemiological Association.

Morbidity = any departure, subjective or objective, from a state of physiological or psychological well-being. (From IEA "A Dictionary of Epidemiology, 1983, Ed. Dr. John Last)

NAPCRG = North American Primary Care Research Group.

Numerator = the number of subjects or items in a study group, used with the denominator to calculate rates

Recorders = participants in a multicentre study, who send data to a central processing unit.

RACGP = The Royal Australian College of General Practitioners

RCGP = The Royal College of General Practitioners (in Britain, from 1962).

Rubrics = numbers identifying items in a classification of diseases.

UWO = University of Western Ontario, also known as 'Western'

WONCA = World Organization of National Colleges and Academies of General Practice/Family Practice and Allied Academic Institutions.

References

Allen, A.B., Barnard, B.G., Falk, W.A., Higgs, E.R., and McCracken, J.G. A Study of Waiting Time in an Emergency Department. CMAJ 1973; 109:373-376.

Andersen, N.L. An Assessment of the Structure of General Practice in New South Wales: Report of a Survey. Med J Aust 1968 2 (suppl):155-167.

A Program of Research. Bull Coll Gen Pract Can 1959; 5(3):23.

Arnold, I.M.F. And Steele, R. Recreational Accidents and the General Practitioners. Can Fam Phys 1968; 14:21-25. (Aug 64 - May 65)

Arnon, A. My Practice in My Pocket. Dept. Of Fam. Med., MUSC,1978.

Baars, C.M. Summary of Emergency Survey at Riverside Hospital, Ottawa. Can Fam Phys 1969; 15:129-133.

Bain, S. and Johnson, S. Use and abuse of Hospital Emergency Departments. Can Fam Phys May 1971; 17:33-36.

Bartel, G.G., Waldie ,A.C., and Rix, D.B. Rural and Urban Family Practice in B.C. - a comparison. Can Fam Phys 1970; 16:121-125.

Baskin, M., Levesque, L., Macpherson, A.S., Poole, P.E., and Sackett. D.L. Canada's Health Care Evaluation Seminars: an Epilogue and Evaluation. Can J Pub Hlth Oct 1980; 71:321-327.

Bass, M. A Profile of Family Practice in London, Ontario. Can Fam Phys 1975; 21:113-120.

Bass, M. The Pharmacist as a provider of primary care. CMAJ 1975(a);112:60-64.

Bass, M. and Copeman, W.J. An Ontario solution to medically underserviced areas: evaluation of an ongoing program. CMAJ 1975(b);113:403-407.

Bentsen, B.G. Illness and General Practice - a survey of medical care in an inland population in Southeast Norway. Universitetsforlaget, Blindern, Oslo 3, 1970.

Black, D.P. Management of myocardial infarction in a rural area. CMAJ 1973;109:863-867.

Black, D.P., Riddle,R.J. and Sampson, E. Pilot project: the family practice nurse in a Newfoundland rural area. CMAJ 1976;114:945-947.

Breinl, W. Preliminary Report on the National Morbidity Survey. Ann Gen Pract 1964; IX:1A, 32.

Bridges-Webb, C. Anaesthetics in General Practice: a Review of 300 Administrations. Med J Austral 1963;2:349.

Bridges-Webb, C. A Study of Morbidity in Traralgon, Victoria (Australia). M.D. Thesis, Monash University, 1971.

Bridges-Webb, C. Survey of Anaesthetics in General Practice in Victoria. Ann Gen Pract 1967; XII:73.

Bridges-Webb, C. A Three-year Study of Respiratory Infections. Annals of General Practice (Convention Proceedings) April 1964; 9(1A):19-31, and Med World 1965;102:381-389.

Brown, D.C. and Yang, K. Childhood Urinary Tract Infections in Family Practice. Can Fam Phys 1972; 18:39-41. (12 months, 690 pts.)

Bury, J.D. The Consumer and Drug Costs. Conference on costs and organization of medical care, Saskatoon Community Health Foundation.
April 18-19,1969.

Canadian Practitioners Invited to Cooperate with British Research Team. Bull Coll Gen Pract Can 1958; 5(2):39.

Cauchon , R. A Coxsackie Epidemic - as seen by a General Practitioner. Bull Coll Gen Pract Can 1960; 7(2):23-25.

Clarke, P.S. Serological (Schulz-Dale) Test for Carcinoma. Med J Austral 1964; 1:315.

Clute, K.F. The General Practitioner. A study of medical education and practice in Ontario and Nova Scotia. University of Toronto Press 1963; (a study of 86 practices, 1956 -1960)

College Members Invited to Conduct Therapeutic Trials on New Pharmaceutical Products. Bull Coll Gen Pract 1959; 6(1):45.

Collier, K.J. One Hundred Vasectomies. Can Fam Phys 1974; 20:57-59.

Collyer, J.A. An Epidemic Influenza Study. Can Fam Phys 1970; 16(2):107-108.

Collyer, J.A. An Evaluation of Treatment in Family Practice. A group research project. Can Fam Phys 1969(b);15(9):44-49.

Collyer, J.A. A Family Doctor's Time. Can Fam Phys 1969(b); 15:63-69.

Collyer, J.A. Psychiatric Care in Family Practice. Can Fam Phys July 1968; 14:44-53.

Collyer, J.A. The Unhappy Fat Woman. Can Fam Phys 1973; 19:93-97.

Comley, A. Family Therapy and the Family Physician. Can Fam Phys Feb 1973; 19:78-81.

Crombie, D.L. and Cross, K.W. The Use of a General Practitioner's Time. Brit J Prev Soc Med 1956; 10:141-144.

Cullen, K.J. A survey of behaviour disorders and related factors in the children of 1,000 Western Australian families. Thesis, Doctorate in Medicine.   Ann Gen Pract 1963;8:216-217.

Cullen, K.J.   A Report on an Investigation of a Country Midwifery Practice, with the Preliminary Results of 300 Cases Following Improved Obstetrical Care.   Med J Austral 1953;2:635-639.

Davies, A.M. Epidemiological Research in General Practice. Expert Committee on General Practice, WHO, 1964.

de Buda. Y.   Investigation of Asymptomatic Proteinuria in Female Patients.   Can Fam Phys 1967;13:31-33.

Dixon, A.S.   Survey of a Rural Practice: Rainy River 1975.   Can Fam Phys 1976(a); 22:693-701, 1976(b);22:963-971.

Eimerl, T.S. Organized Curiosity: A practical approach to the problem of keeping records for research purposes in general practice.   J Coll Gen Practit 1960; 3:246-52.

Eimerl, T.S. and Laidlaw, A.J.. A Handbook for Research in General Practice. E. & S. Livingstone Ltd, Edinburgh and London, 1969.

Elford, R.W. The "E Book" Turned Chronic Illness Register. Can Fam Phys 1975; 21:35-37.

Falk, W.A. Research News Page: Can Fam Phys Jan 1974; 41.

Falk, W.A. Detailed Study of a Practice Population and its Illness. National Health Grant 609-7-260.   1971:unpublished.

Fallis, F.   Metro Toronto G.P.'s - who, where, how many?   Can Fam Phys 1971;17:33-39. (690 in 1968)

Fowler, J.A. and Falk, W.A.   A Study of GP Hospital Admissions in B.C. Can Fam Phys June 1973; 56-59.

Fry, J. A Year of General Practice: A Study in Morbidity. Brit Med J 1952; 249-252.

Fry, J. and Blake, P. Keeping of Records in General Practice. Brit Med J 1 (suppl) 1956: 339-341.

Fry, J. Five Years of General Practice: A Study in Simple Epidemiology.   Brit Med J 1957; 1453-1457.

Fry, J. Profiles of Disease. A Study in the Natural History of Diseases. Williams and Wilkins, Baltimore, 1966.

Fry, J. and Dillane, J.B. Too Much Work? Proposals Based on a Review of Fifteen Years' Work in Practice.   Lancet 1964;632-634.

Gallagher, D.J.A., Montgomerie, J.Z. and North,J.D.K . Acute Infections of the Urinary Tract and the Urethral Syndrome in General Practice.   Brit Med J 1965;(1)622-626.

Garson. J. Z. A Weekend on Call in Canada. J.Roy Coll Gen Practit 1973; 23:293-296.

Garson, J.Z. Check-ups - useful or useless?   Conference on costs and organization of medical care. Saskatoon Community Health Foundation, April 18-19, 1969.

Garson, J.Z., Boor, S., McAskill, J., Altwasser, M.,and Loraas, S. The check-up centre as part of an ongoing medical practice.   Can Fam Phys 1972;18:93-100. (6 months, 273 charts).

Garson, J.Z. and Wolfe, R.R.   Social Problems of the Hospitalized Elderly. Can Fam Phys Nov 1975;21:85-93.

Ghan, L. and Road, D. Social Work in a Mixed Group Medical Practice. Can J Pub Health 1970; 61:488-496.

Gibson, W.C.   1978. Personal communication, Woodward Library, the University of British Columbia.

Greenhill, S. and Atkinson, M. A Critical Evaluation of a Family Study Program. J Coll Gen Pract Can 1964; 10:22-23.

140

Greenhill, S. and Kolotyluk, K. The Hospital Bed and the General Practitioner: a pilot study of two practices with respect to hospital bed usage and patient management. Can Med Assn J 1965; 93:67-72.

Greenhill, S. and Singh, H.J. Comparisons of the Functions of Medical Practitioners in Rural Areas with those in Urban Areas. J Med Educ 1964; 39:806-809.

Greenhill, S. and Singh, H.J. Comparisons of the Professional Functions of Rural and Urban Practitioners. J Med Educ 1965; 40:856-865.

Greenhill, S. and Watts, P. Some Differences between Patients seen in Practitioners' Offices and those Admitted to Teaching Hospitals: an exploratory study. J Med Educ 1964; 39: 1228-1231.

Gretton, A.H. Alberta Mental Health Study. Can Fam Phys Nov 1968;14:49-56.

Hammond, M. Research Projects by General Practitioners, Second Edition Revised. Royal College of General Practitioners, London, 1971.

Hart, W.J. Streptococcal Pharyngitis. Can Fam Phys 1976;22:516-521.

Heaton, P. The Diagnostic Problem of Prescribing Antibiotics in URI. Can Fam Phys 1973; 19:55-58.

Heaton, P. and Flett, D. The Doctor and the Community Health Nurse. Can Fam Phys 1971; 17:71-79. (25 consecutive referrals)

Hebb, M. Et al. Nova Scotia Fetal Risk Project. Can Fam Phys Dec 1980; 26:1664-1673.

Hill, A. B. Principles of Medical Statistics. (Seventh Edition) Oxford University Press, New York, 1961.

Hill, M., McAuley, R.G., Spaulding, W.B. and Wilson, M. Validity of the Term "Family Doctor": a Limited Study in Hamilton, Ontario. CMAJ 1968;98:734-738.

Hodgkin, Keith. Towards Earlier Diagnosis. E. & S. Livingston Ltd., Edinburgh and London, 1963.

Hope-Simpson. R.E. Studies on Shingles (is the virus ordinary chickenpox virus?). Lancet 1954; 2:1299-1302.

Hope-Simpson, R.E. The Nature of Herpes Zoster: a long-term study and a new hypothesis. Proc Roy Soc Med 1965; 58:9-20.

Hopkinson, M.A. & Hopkinson, N.E.J.   The General Practitioner Looks at Elevated Blood Pressure. J Coll Gen Pract 1961; 7(6):32-41.

Horder, J. and Horder, E. Illness in General Practice. The Practitioner. Aug 1954;173:177-187.

Hunter, A. T. and Clark, M. The Work of Nurses in a Family Medical Centre. Can Fam Phys 1971; 17:37-41. (4 nurses, 3 weeks)

International Classification of Health Problems in Primary Care. Classification Committee of WONCA; American Hosp Assoc 1975.

Jungfer, C. General Practice in Australia. A report on a survey. Annals of Gen Pract (Aust) March 1965; 4-48.

Kuenssberg, E.V. Recording the morbidity of families. "F" book. J Coll Gen Practit 1964; 7:410-422.

Labelle, C. Alberta Workload Study. Can Fam Phys 1973;19:100-103.

Lane, R.F. A Cervical Cytology Program in General Practice. Can Med Assn J 1965; 92:1203-6.

Lawee, D. An Evaluation of 1,000 Serum Calcium and Inorganic Phosphate Determinations. Can Fam Phys 1970; 16(12):57-60.

le Riche, W.H. Research in Family Practice: let's ask the right questions. Can Fam Phys Feb 1975; 21:52-61.

Livingston, M.C.P. The Background of some Canadian general practitioner observers. Can Med Assn J Apr 1972; 106:797-799.

Livingston, M.C.P. Research and the Canadian Practitioner. The Practitioner 1971; 206:675-680.

Livingston, M.C.P. Researching Recent Researchers. Can Fam Phys May 1974;20:84.

Livingston, M.C.P. Spinal Manipulation: a one-year follow-up study. Can Fam Phys 1969;15:35-38. (60 pts)

Last,J.M. and White, K.L. The Content of Medical Care in Primary Practice. Med Care 1969; 7:41-48.

Loftus, P. The House Call: a Descriptive Study. Can Fam Phys 1976;22:1243-1251.

MacFarlane, A.H. and O'Connell, B.P. Morbidity in Family Practice. Can Med Assn J. 1969; 101:259-263. (12 months, 3005 contacts)

Macpherson, I.G., Fraser, J. and Nurse, E.G. Research in Family Practice: Its Development in Nova Scotia. The N.S. Med Bull June 1970; 49(4):107-109.

Marshall, E.J. Morbidity Recording for Research. N. Z. Med J. 1963;62:484-485.

McKenzie, C. Why Do Doctors Remain in General Practice?

McKenzie, J. The Principles of Diagnosis and Treatment in Heart Affections. Edn. 1916, 1923, 1926.

McQuitty, G.D.H. The Proper Study of Family Practice. Can Fam Phys Sept 1973; 19:113-115.

McWhinney, I.R. The Early Diagnosis of Cancer. J Coll Gen Pract 1962; 5:404-414.

McWhinney, I.R. The Early Signs of Illness. 1964. Charles C. Thomas - Publisher, Springfield, Illinois, USA.

Medalie, J.H. Family Medicine - Principles and Applications. The Williams and Wilkins Company, Baltimore, 1978.

Morgan, R.W., Mansfield, P.J. Geographic Distribution and availability of Physicians in Vancouver. Can Fam Phys 1969; 15(11): 123-127.

Morrison, C.S. Chloroquine as an anti-inflammatory Agent. Research Newsletter, New Zealand Council of General Practitioners 1963; 4:4-7.

Murray, J.V. Obstetrical Experience of a General Practitioner. Bull Coll Gen Pract 1959; 6(3):21 (Reported in B.C. Medical Journal)

Newfoundland Chapter, the College of Family Physicians of Canada. A Transatlantic Morbidity Study. Can Fam Phys 1969; 15:133-140.

Pacy, H. Road Accidents: the Medical Rescuer. Med J Aust 1967; 1:806-809.

Pacy, H. Holiday Hazards. Med J Austral 1961,ii;1010-1015.

Partington M.W., and Anderson, R.M. College of General Practice of Canada. Case-finding in Phenylketonuria. Report of a survey by the College of General Practice of Canada. Can Med Assn J 1964; 90:1312-14.

Pawlowski, G.J. Indomethacin in Traumatic Musculo-skeletal Disorders. Can Fam Phys 1971; 17:93-99. (100 pts.)

Pemberton, J. Will Pickles of Wensleydale. London, Geoffrey Bles, 1970.

Pickles, W.N. Epidemiology in a Country Practice. Bristol, John Wright and Sons, 1939 (re-issued 1949).

Pickles, W.N. Epidemic Catarrhal Jaundice. Lancet 1939(1); 893.

Pinsent, R.J.F.H. The Evolving Age-sex Register. J Roy Coll Gen Practit 1968;16:127-134.

Postuk, P.D., Coleman, J.U., and MacKenzie, C.J.G. An Analysis of the Practice of Four Physicians in British Columbia. Can Fam Phys 1969; 15(1): 51-57.

Postuk, P.D. and Mackenzie, C.J.G. A report of an analysis of general practice in British Columbia from a study of the practices of 54 physicians - 1964. Unpublished manuscript.

Radford, J.G. Morbidity recording in one year of general practice. Part I
Ann Gen Pract 1963;8:134-142. Part II - Ann Gen Pract 1964;9:98-105.

Rhodes, A.J. In "G.P.'s collect data on Echo Virus 9". Bull Coll Gen Pract Can 1957; 4(2):16.

Records and Statistics Unit, College of General Practitioners: Some Contrasts in Morbidity Distribution. J Coll Gen Practit 1966; 11:74-83.

Research Digest. The Australian College of General Practitioners. Vol. 1, 1968

Ross, J. A Study of Morbidity in Family Practice. Can Fam Phys 1972; 18:105-115. (6 rural Practices, 18 months)

Rosser, W.W. and Flett, D.E. How Patients Follow Hospital Discharge Instructions in an Urban Family Practice. Can Fam Phys 1971; 17:57-59., (23 patients)

Rowe, I.L., editor. Research Digest, The Australian College of General Practitioners, Vol 1, 1958-1968; Vol 2, 1972.

Rowe, I.L. Postpartum Hemorrhage in Relation to Methods of Management of Labour. Med J Austral 1962;1:109-116.

Rudnick, K.V. Screening for Hypertension: Case-finding. Can Fam Phys 1979;25:1170-1172.

Rudnick, K.V., Spitzer, W.O., and Pierce, J. Comparison of a Private Family Practice and a University Teaching Centre. J Med Educ 1976; 51:395-402.

Rutter, P. Myocardial Infarction in a Canadian Rural Practice. Can Fam Phys 74; 20:67-68.

Sackett, D.L., Baskin, M.S. ed. Methods of Health Care Evaluation – Readings and Exercises developed for the National Health Grant Health Care Evaluation Seminars. 1971 (third edition 1978).

Shardt, A. The Family Practitioner in a Multi-specialty Group: Obstetrics. Can Fam Phys 1970;16:60-63. (1960-1969 stats, 722 pts.)

Shardt, A. The Family Practitioner in a Multi-specialty Group: Patterns of Practice. Can Fam Phys 1969; 15:51-55. (6 mos. work)

Shardt, A. The Family Practitioner in a Multi-specialty Group: Special Services. Can Fam Phys 1971;17:58-60.

Shephard, D.A.E. A Light on Medical Practice in 19th Century Canada; the medical manuscripts of Dr. John Mackieson of Charlottetown. Can Med Assoc J 1998; 159(3):253-257.

Sibley, J.C., Spitzer, W.O., Rudnick, K.V., Bell, J.D., Bethune, R.D., Sackett, D.L. and Wright, K. Quality –of –Care Appraisal in Primary Care: a Quantitative Method. Ann Int Med 1975; 83:46-52.

Simms, J.G. and Rosser, W.W. Farmer's Lung in Urbanites. Can Fam Phys 1971 16:69-71. (37 pts.)

Staines, F.H and Forman, J.A.S. A Survey of Farmer's Lung.
J Coll Gen Pract 1961; 4:351-382.

Staples, J.C. The Use of Haldol in Obstetrics. Can Fam Phys 1967; 13(10): 23-25.

Steele, R., Kraus, A.S. and Smith, P.M. Doctor/patient Contacts in Family Practice. An exploratory Study, Can Fam Phys 1968;14:45-55. (1-week period 1966)

Sweeney, G.P. and Hay, W.I. The Burlington Experience: a Study of Nurse Practitioners in Family Practice. Can Fam Phys Sept 1973; 101-110.

Taylor, J.A. The Working Hours of a General Practitioner. Can Fam Phys 1968; 14:43-47. (Workload, July-Dec 1967)

Teglas, A.L. Patterns of Emergency Practice. Can Fam Phys Oct 1969;15:56-59.

Tenney, J.B. The Content of Medical Practice - a research bibliography. April 1969. Department of Medical Care and Hospitals, Johns Hopkins University.

Thomson, A. McQ. Unexpected findings at routine Examinations. Ann Gen Pract 1971; XVI:79.

Thomson, A. McQ. Cancer Detection is Practical. Med J Austral 1958; 1:699.

A Transatlantic Morbidity Study - a joint research project between the Newfoundland Chapter of the College of Family Physicians of Canada and the Research Unit of the Royal College of General Practitioners, Great Britain. Can Fam Phys Sept 69;15:133-140, also J Coll Gen Practit 1969; 18:137-147.

Trenholme, M. Women Doctors in Family Practice. Can Fam Phys 1967; Part 1: 13(9):45-55. Part 2: 13(10):37-44.

Valentine, A.S. What is Family Practice? Maybe the E Book can tell you. Can Fam Phys 1975; 21:29-35.

Waldie, A.C. and Rix, D.B. Comparison of Pattern and Range of Practice of a three-man group in a large city with that of a similar group in a small town (see Bartel, above).

Warner, M.M. Family Medicine in a Consumer Age. Monograph 1975; prepared for the Lay Advisory and Research Committee of the College of Family Physicians of Canada, B.C. Chapter.

Warner, M.M. Family Medicine in a Consumer Age. Can Fam Phys 1977; 23:   Part 1: The Mechanics of Care, p. 569...
        Part 2: The Doctor/Patient Relationship and Social Problems, p.706...
        Part 3: Family Physicians and Other Health Professionals, p.809...
        Part 4: Preventive Medicine, Professional Satisfaction, and the Rise of Consumerism, p. 925...

West, S.R. When is the Baby Due? NZ Med J 1965;64:282-284.

Westbury, R.C. Research Awareness Publication. Can Fam Phys March 1971; 17:77.

Westbury. R.C. RAPid Entry into the World of Family Medicine Research. Can Fam Phys May 1973; 19:111.

Westbury, R.C. The National Library of Family Medicine. Can Fam Phys 1970; 16:97-101.

Westbury, R.C. and Tarrant M. Classification of Disease in General Practice: a comparative study. Can Med Assn J.; 101:603-608.

Westbury, R.C. The Electric Speaking Practice: a telephone workload study. Can Fam Phys 1974; 20:69-72.

Weston, W. Beyond the Scribbled Note. Can Fam Phys May 1973; 19:83-90.

White, K.L. et al. The Ecology of Medical Care. NEJM 1961; 265(18):885-892.

White, K.L. Family Medicine, Academic Medicine, and the University's Responsibility. JAMA 1963 July 20; 185:192-196.

Williams, W.O. A cheap and simple method of recording sudden epidemics. Between Ourselves 1964;23:6-7.

Williams, W.O. A Study of General Practitioners' Workload in South Wales. 1965-66. RCGP Reports from general practice No. 12; January 1970.

Wolfe, S., Badgley, R.F., Kasius, R.V., Garson, J.Z. and Gold, R.J.M. The Work of a Group of Doctors in Saskatchewan, Milbank Mem Fund Q Jan 1968;46(1):103-130.

Wolfe, S., and Badgley, R.F. The Family Doctor. Milbank Mem Fund Q April 1972;50(2):1-203.

Woods, D. Strength in Study. An informal history of the College of Family Physicians of Canada. 1979, published by the College.

Workman, D.G. and Cunningham, D.G. Effect of Psychotropic Drugs on Aggression in a Prison Setting. Can Fam Phys 1975; 21:63-66.

Wright, G.L.T. The Queensland Asthma Survey.. Annals of General Practice April 1964; 9(1A):7-18.

Wright, H.J. - Reports from General Practice. VIII General Practice in Southwest England. The Royal College of General Practitioners, 1968.

Zabarenko, L. & Zwell, E. Bibliography - Research in General Practice. Staunton Clinic, Western Psychiatric Institute and Clinic, School of Medicine, U. Of Pittsburgh, 1968.

Zack, J.J. Service in the Emergency Department of the Vancouver General Hospital by the Department of General Practice. J Coll Gen Pract 1967; 13(5): 39-45.

Zwell M.E. and Zaborenko, L. Training for Family Practice, a selected bibliography. Staunton Clinic, Western Psychiatric Institute and Clinic, School of Medicine, U. of Pittsburgh, 1970.

Index

Fairley, H., 62,122
Falk,W.A.,45,46,,58,61,62,65,
121,122,125-127,129-131,134
Fallis, F., 36
Farquhar, D., 108
Ferguson, D.C., 127,128
Fern, B., 128
Fish, D.G., 57
Fitsgerald, D., 86
Fletcher, H.G., 53
Flett, D., 132
Forgiel, C., 126
Foster, W., 4
Fowler, J.A., 45,58,106
Fraser, B., 134
Fraser, J., 64
Fraser, W.R., 52
Froom, J., 72,130
Fry, J., 8,100,131
Gallagher, D.J.A., 16
Game, D., 17
Garson, J.Z., 30,34,41,43,44,62,
63,65,92,111,114,122,125,127,
129,134
Garson, R., 63,93
Gay, K.E., 59,122
Ghan, L., 35
Gibson, G.,79
Gibson, M., 78
Gibson, W.C., 26
Gillis, W.R., 126
Glick, D., 126
Gooderham, M.E.W., 50
Gordon, C., 16
Gowdy, C.W., 60
Greenhill, S., 55,56,57,80
Geller, K.G., 58
Gretton, A.H., 35,126
Haines, M., 60
Hall, B., 60
Hamilton, G., 53
Hammond, M., 80,87
Harrison, R.C., 57
Hart, W.J., 40
Heaton, P., 33,123,126
Hebb, A.M., 116,126,128,129,131
Hibbard, R., 133
Hilditch, J., 126

Hill, A.B., 109
Hodgkin, K., 9,64,131,134
Hogben, 109
Hole, L., 134
Hollenberg, H.J., 60
Hoogewerf, P., 63
Hope-Simpson, E., 8
Hopkinson, M.A.,28
Hopkinson, N.E.J., 28
Horders, 8
Horne, J., 134
Hunter, R.C.A., 55
Hunter, A.T., 59,122
Hutchinson, 11
Hutchison, D.A., 56,59
Huygen, 10
Irwin, D., 123
Jeffrey, E.S., 52,53
Johnson, A., 86
Johnston, M., 133
Johnston, W.V., 52
Jungfer, C., 3,13
Kapos, A., 123
Karpilow, C., 133
Kay, C., 70,125,126
Kedworth, H., 123
Keeting, M., 126
Keith, W.D., 26
Kling, S., 56
Knapp, J.E., 123
Kolotyluk, K., 55
Kraus, A., 132
Krause, R., 59
Kuenssberg, E., 70,100,107,
125, 126
Labelle, C., 41,65,126
Laidlaw, A.J., 102
Lamont, C., 59,122
Lane, R.F., 27
Lang, S., 123
Last, J.M., 73,116,132
Laszlo, C., 83,134
Lawee, D., 37,122,131
le Riche, H., 80,127,128
Lewis, R.,56
Librach, S., 133
Livingston, M., ix,37,85
Lloyd, G., 55
Loftus, P., 43

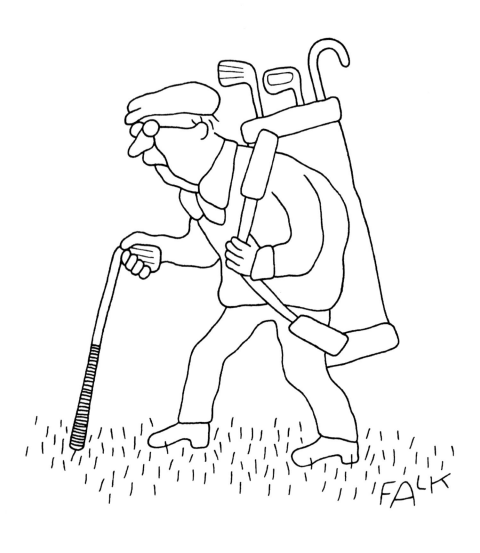

ISBN 155212777-X